"In *The Most Effective Natural Cures on Earth*, you'll find literally hundreds of proven, natural solutions—many of which I use in my own practice. This book is a must-have reference for anyone interested in discovering the natural options that really work."

—**Al Sears, M.D.,** author of *The Doctor's Heart Cure*

"This book is a must for everyone's library. I think of this book as natural first aid."

—**Shari Lieberman, Ph.D., C.N.S., F.A.C.N.,** author of *The Gluten Connection*, and Founding Dean of New York Chiropractic Colleges' Masters of Science Program in Applied Clinical Nutrition

"Jonny Bowden has once again dug deep into the science, finding the best available natural treatments for the most common ailments."

—**Mark Hyman, M.D.,** author of *UltraMetabolism* and *The UltraSimple Diet* and Founder and Medical Director of The UltraWellness Center

"This is an excellent, user-friendly book that skillfully guides you through the maze of natural health solutions. It's thorough, well-written, and research-based."

—**Hyla Cass, M.D.,** Assistant Clinical Professor of Psychiatry at UCLA School of Medicine and author of *Supplement Your Prescription*

"When it comes to putting together nutritional programs that people can see and feel the difference, Bowden not only has the experience but has also the technical knowledge to make it happen."

—**Stephen T. Sinatra, M.D., F.A.C.C., F.A.C.N., C.N.S.,** Cardiologist and coauthor, *Reverse Heart Disease Now*

"An empowering experience for anyone wanting to take charge of their own health!"

—**Daniel G. Amen, M.D.,** author of *Healing ADD* and *Change Your Brain, Change Your Life* and a Distinguished Fellow of the American Psychiatric Association

"Well done! Get ready to be empowered to reclaim control of your health and well-being!"

—**Jacob Teitelbaum M.D.,** author of *From Fatigued to Fantastic!* Medical Director, the Fibromyalgia and Fatigue Centers

"Another must-read from Jonny Bowden. Highly recommended!"

—**Dharma Singh Khalsa, M.D.,** author of *Meditation As Medicine* and Director of the Alzheimer's Prevention Foundation International

"This book should be the first place to look before calling your doctor. Every household in America needs at least one of this great reference manual to a healthy life, naturally."

—**Fred Pescatore, M.D., M.P.H., C.C.N.,** author of the *New York Times* bestseller, *The Hamptons Diet*

The Most Effective Natural Cures on Earth

The Surprising, Unbiased Truth
about What Treatments Work and Why

Jonny Bowden, Ph.D., C.N.S.

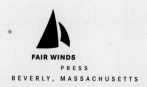

FAIR WINDS
PRESS
BEVERLY, MASSACHUSETTS

© 2011 Fair Winds Press
Text © 2008, 2011 Jonny Bowden
This edition published in 2011

First published in the USA in 2008 by
Fair Winds Press, a member of
Quayside Publishing Group
100 Cummings Center
Suite 406-L
Beverly, Massachusetts 01915-6101
www.fairwindspress.com

15 14 13 12 11 1 2 3 4 5

ISBN-13: 978-59233-474-2
ISBN-10: 1-59233-474-1

Originally under the following Library of Congress Cataloging-in-Publication Data

Bowden, Jonny.
   The most effective natural cures on earth : what treatments work
and why / Jonny Bowden.
      p. cm.
   Includes index.
   ISBN-13: 978-1-59233-291-5
   ISBN-10: 1-59233-291-9
   1. Naturopathy. 2. Alternative medicine. I. Title.
RZ440.B645 2008
615.5'35--dc22
                                        2007035953
                                        CIP

Cover design: Dutton and Sherman Design
Book production: Megan Cooney
Photography: Glenn Scott Photography

Printed and bound in China

The information in this book is for educational purposes only. It is not intended to replace the
advice of a physician or medical practitioner. Please see your health-care provider before beginning
any new health program.

Fair Winds Press would like to thank Conley's pharmacy of Ipswich, Massachusetts,
for its generosity and assistance in helping with the photos for this book.

Pill sizes, shapes, and colors may vary among manufacturers.

To Anja

Who, for me, makes almost anything possible

"The natural healing force within each of us is the greatest force in getting well."

—Hippocrates

"Western medicine doesn't hold all the answers. Healing cannot always be described in numbers."

—Mehmet C. Oz, M.D.

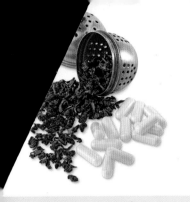
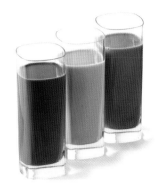
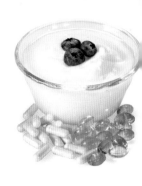

CONTENTS

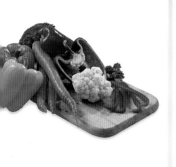
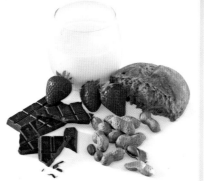
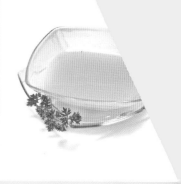

INTRODUCTION

L et me be perfectly honest with you—*Natural Cures* was not, at first, my favorite title for this book.

"Cure" is a word I don't like to use when talking about natural treatments. Natural medicine—or nutritional medicine—works by treating the whole body as a system. It's not a philosophy based on taking a pill to suppress a symptom; it's about healing the condition that caused the symptom in the first place. And this generally involves an entire prescription for healing that can be as simple as a taking a few vitamins, but more typically, combines lifestyle, nutritional, physical, psychological, and even spiritual components, not your conventional "cure."

I also don't want to denigrate the power and usefulness of nutritional medicine by opening myself up to charges of hucksterism, so let me be perfectly clear from the outset: A vitamin doesn't "cure" cancer. A mineral doesn't "cure" diabetes, and there's no "natural cure" for Alzheimer's. These are serious conditions with many overlapping facets and problems, and they can't be "cured" by a pill.

However, a big "but" goes with that disclaimer.

The natural treatments in this book—vitamins, herbs, minerals, foods, plants, or any of the many specific treatments or combinations of compounds—can make a huge difference in your health. No kidding. They can address certain metabolic conditions and blocked pathways that can contribute to your illness.

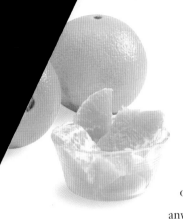

They can clear up some of the obstacles that stand in the way of your healing. They can jump-start the body's amazing, natural curative powers. In some cases, following these prescriptions can actually "cure" a condition, or at least make it so minor that it doesn't bother you anymore. In some cases, they may not completely eliminate the condition, but you may find that you're able to significantly reduce your dependence on medication. In still other cases, they may give you a partial improvement and relieve a good portion of your suffering.

BODY, HEAL THYSELF

Natural medicine—in fact, all traditional systems of healing from traditional Chinese medicine to shamanism to herbalism—subscribe to a basic philosophy that seems to be curiously absent in conventional Western medicine, and it's this: The body has an almost wondrous ability to heal itself. My friend, naturopathic physician Sonja Petterson, N.M.D., points out that in sanatoriums they used to put people on fasts, hose them down, and make them walk around in the cold clean air. It sounds barbaric, and it probably was, but the philosophy behind it—now long lost in high-tech medicine—was to get patients to rally their bodies' own amazing resources and capacity for healing.

"My best friend in med school was a vet," Petterson says, "and that's what they always do when an animal is sick. They withdraw food and let them sleep. That's what an animal does in the wild, and that's what your dog does if he's sick. He stops eating and sleeps a lot. He instinctively knows that's what it takes to heal."

As in many areas of life, we can learn a lot from our dogs.

The lesson here is that your body has a natural tendency to heal itself, a fact that many of us seem to have forgotten. Natural medicine simply helps that process along. Nourish your body with the nutrients it needs to perform the metabolic processes involved in getting rid of viruses, bacteria, and other toxins. Support its immune responses. Stop overwhelming it with poisons, bad food, stress, polluted air, and toxic relationships. Allow it plenty of time to sleep and repair. Give it some sunshine and, yup, some tender loving.

Sound granola-ish? Maybe. But if that's one extreme approach to healing and the other end of the spectrum is heavy medication for symptoms, maybe we could look for something that's a little more of a compromise. Maybe we could begin to take advantage of the body's own miraculous ability to repair and heal by giving it natural substances that support it in that journey. And that, in a nutshell, is the purpose of this book.

HOW NATURAL CURES HELP YOU

One of my friends, Joseph Brasco, M.D.—interviewed for this book for his expertise in all things gastrointestinal—told me about his "rule of thirds," something that applies to the majority of the natural treatments and "cures" I write about in this book.

"One-third of the people I treat with natural medicine [like diet and supplements] will get 100 percent better—effectively cured," he told me. "One-third will improve considerably—they may be able to go off meds, or reduce meds substantially, or their symptoms will lessen, or they'll have measurably less pain and suffering. And one-third, unfortunately, won't be helped very much at all."

I agree with this, but I'd go one step further. Even for the one-third of the population whose condition might not be terribly responsive to a given treatment or "cure," chances are that some area of their health will be or could be improved by following the natural prescription for their condition outlined in this book. And that could make a big difference in their overall well-being.

For example, the Paleo Diet might not entirely clear up acne in every single person who has acne, but it will almost always have an important positive effect on blood sugar and weight. And while the "kidney stone cure" of magnesium and vitamin B6 might not relieve every single case of kidney stones, the ingredients in it work together in dozens of ways in the body to improve mood and well-being. And omega-3 fatty acids, which are a part of a number of cures, have a positive effect on so many areas of health and well-being that it's hard to imagine how anyone on the planet wouldn't benefit from them.

So the "cures" in this book will never hurt anyone, and I like to think they will help most people—at least a little, if not substantially. Best of all, not one ingredient in any of the "cures" is addictive, and not one of them has the remotest potential for abuse or for death by overdose. Though it's certainly possible to take a "toxic" dose of a vitamin or herb (just as it's theoretically possible to have a "toxic" overdose of water) in real life, it's just not very likely. The "cures" in this book present substantially less risk to your health than prescription medications do, and the likelihood of any negative side effects from any of the natural prescriptions listed in this book—taken as directed—are incredibly small.

Remember, though, this is not "faith healing." You're not going to throw away your crutches in a single moment and proclaim, "I'm healed, I can walk again!" and go skipping out of the revival tent. No, in that narrow sense, the treatments and prescriptions in this book are not technically "cures." But they sure are powerful helpmates on your road to health. And they may feel like lifesavers to a lot of people. For everyone else, they will get you healthier, and they will make a difference.

And I'm pretty sure that, for some folks, they will make all the difference in the world.

WHY THIS BOOK IS DIFFERENT

If there's one thing that sets *The Most Effective Natural Cures on Earth* apart from the spate of other "natural cure" books it's this: research.

Let me explain. The major objection the average person is likely to hear from establishment doctors about "natural medicine" is that there's "no good research showing it works." We hear this constantly about vitamins, antioxidants, herbs, and all sorts of non-medical healing traditions (from acupuncture to shamanism). (Later I'll go into why we hear this refrain constantly and the reason the media tends to report on vitamin studies so negatively.)

The point is that it's not true.

There's a ton of research on vitamins, minerals, phytochemicals, amino acids, fatty acids, and other nutritive substances. (Want proof? Go to the National Library of Medicine/National Institutes of Health online library, www.pubmed.gov, and put any vitamin you can think of in the search engine.) The problem isn't that there's an absence of research—it's that a great deal of this research flies under the radar screen of those whom we turn to for health advice.

But the research exists. I've found it, you can find it, and your doctor can find it. You just have to be open to looking at it. You'll find dozens and dozens of references to published studies throughout the text of this book.

Now let me be fully frank—I wish the research were more definitive. But research in vitamins and minerals and other "natural" substances doesn't lend itself to the same kind of design as research on drugs, and therein may be one of the many problems with getting this information out there. We're used to having a symptom, taking a drug, and seeing the symptom disappear. Nutrients work differently. For one thing, they generally work in combination, much like the way they're found in nature. For another, they work more slowly and more subtly, repairing the mechanisms that caused the symptom in the first place. But that said, the substantial research on the vast majority of ingredients in this book should cause even the greatest skeptic to consider the possibilities that these non-invasive, gentle treatments could help heal a vast array of conditions and bring health to a vast number of people.

THE GOAL OF THIS BOOK

My goal in this book—and, come to think of it, every book I've ever written—is to empower you. It's to help you become not only an active participant in your own health care, but the leader of your own health-care team. I want you to be captain of Team You. I don't want you to follow me—or any other "'guru'" of health—but rather learn to listen with open heart and mind, try things on, see whether they work, use what does, and throw away what doesn't.

Back in the 1990s when I was working as a personal trainer in New York City, gyms were springing up all over the city. The *New York Times* called the phenomenon "The Gym Wars." There was much discussion about where to go to get the best workout, about who had the best aerobics classes, about which location had the most state-of-the-art equipment, which gym had the best trainers, and so on. I remember being interviewed at the time by one of the magazines, and being asked, "Which gym is best?"

Here was my answer: The best gym is the one you actually go to.

I was reminded of this exchange when I was talking to Walter Bortz, M.D., a faculty member at Stanford, the author of *Dare to Be 100*, and the president of a great organization called Fifty-Plus Lifelong Fitness. He's also seventy years old and runs at least one marathon a year. We were talking about exercise and I asked him, as a master's athlete, doctor, and lifelong fitness advocate: What's the best kind of exercise, all things considered?

Here was his answer: The best exercise in the world is the exercise you actually do. I think the germ of truth in both these answers—mine and Bortz's—can be applied to natural cures and healing in general. The best treatment is the one that actually works for you. In the long run, you are in charge of your health. Listen wisely to those you trust, but ultimately make your own decisions. Remember that your health is both a gift that was given to you and a gift that you give the world. When you are not healthy—when you are less than your best—when you are living, as William James said, "a life inferior to ourselves," you are depriving me and everyone else of the enormous contribution you have to make to the world.

You owe it to yourself and to me and to everyone else around you to be the fullest expression of who you are. That means a healthy body, mind, and spirit. Don't settle for less.

Enjoy the journey.

Acne

Clear Up This Condition with the Paleo Diet and Saw Palmetto

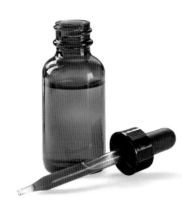

TELL JOHN MCDOUGALL that acne has nothing to do with diet and be prepared to see him fighting mad. "Next time you hear that, ask for the evidence," he says.

McDougall, medical director of the renowned McDougall Wellness Center in Santa Rosa, California, traces this wrongheaded information to a seriously flawed study by James Fulton, M.D., in the *Journal of the American Medical Association* way back in 1969. Fulton, aided by the Chocolate Manufacturers Association of America, tested thirty adolescents and thirty-five young adult male prisoners. He gave the subjects one of two sugar- and fat-loaded candy bars—one with and one without chocolate. Then, at the end of the study, he counted their pimples. The complexions of forty-six of the sixty-five subjects stayed the same, ten actually improved, and nine showed more acne. Based on this highly suspect and flawed study, the claim that "diet has nothing to do with acne" was born and remains the conventional wisdom to this day.

Opposing Forces Create Confusion

I hate to be cynical, but one reason that doctors and dermatologists say that diet doesn't cause acne is because they can't sell a healthy diet. In addition, they were trained to believe that there's no connection between what you eat and what your face looks like. Plus, there's constant pressure from the pharmaceutical industry to prescribe creams, drugs, and other "remedies."

The problem is muddied further by the fact that there isn't a perfect correlation between diet and acne—some people can eat crap all day long and have perfect skin and others can eat healthfully and still have outbreaks. "Acne sufferers are not a homogenous group," says Richard Fried, M.D., Ph.D., author of *Healing Adult Acne*.

Two events conspire to create or aggravate most forms of acne. One is blockage, two is infection. Here's how it works: Keratin is a fibrous protein that's the main component of the outermost layer of the skin. Sebum is part of the oil found on the surface of the skin and is produced by the sebaceous glands, most of which open into a hair follicle. When either too much keratin or sebum is produced, it can block the skin pores. Those overstuffed pores then can become infected by bacteria, which literally eat up the sebum and thrive.

There is overwhelming evidence—both clinical and theoretical—that diet is a huge contributor to acne. Skeptical? Then ponder this: if diet has nothing to do with acne, why is the incidence of acne in underdeveloped countries where people eat natural, native diets almost zero while the incidence of acne in Western countries is in the double digits?

Eating Locally and Healthfully

The idea that the Western diet has nothing to do with acne should have been given its walking papers years ago. Back in 1971, O. Schaeffer published a report that acne was completely absent in the Inuit (Eskimo) population when they were eating and living in their traditional manner, but as soon as they adopted the Western way of eating, acne showed up.

Local physicians in Okinawa prior to World War II reported that "These people had no acne vulgaris." According to one report, only 2.7 percent of almost 10,000 rural Brazilian school kids have acne. There's far less acne in Kenya, Zambia, Malaysia, and rural Japan than is common in Western societies.

But if there was any doubt left about the diet-acne connection it should have been erased by the seminal research paper published in the Archives of Dermatology in 2002 by respected researcher Loren Cordain, Ph.D., of Colorado State University.

Cordain and his team studied two non-Westernized populations: the Kitavan Islanders of Papua New Guinea and the Ache hunter-gatherers of Paraguay. Are you ready for the number of cases of acne observed by these trained researchers?

None. Of 1,200 Kitavan subjects and 115 Ache subjects examined, not a single case of active acne was observed.

Tubers, fruit, fish, and coconut represent the dietary mainstays in Kitava and, according to Cordain, dietary habits are virtually uninfluenced by Western foods in most households. Similarly, the diet of the Ache of eastern Paraguay contains wild, foraged foods, locally grown foods, and only about 8 percent Western foods.

Ancestral Advantages

In other words, they were eating the diet of our hunter-gatherer ancestors: food you could hunt, gather, pluck, or fish, what Cordain, author of a well-respected book by the same name, calls *The Paleo Diet*. In another of his books, *The Dietary Cure for Acne*, he lays out some tasty options for a diet based on whole foods—salmon, sirloin, strawberries, walnuts, carrots, and the like—which may well be the cornerstone of a natural prescription for getting rid of acne. (The paleo diet is absent of grains and dairy and high in grass-fed meats, vegetables, fruits, and omega fats.)

Cordain hypothesizes that a diet that produces high levels of the hormone insulin is partly the culprit when it comes to acne. Here's how it works: High-sugar foods (processed carbs and the like) produce higher levels of a hormone called insulin, which in turn elicits a rise in another hormone called IGF-1 (Insulin-like growth factor). IGF-1 has a high potential for stimulating growth in all tissues, including the follicles. Both insulin and IGF-1 stimulate more hormones in both ovarian and testicular tissues, meaning they stimulate more testosterone (in both men and women). And more testosterone—with its especially nasty metabolite DHT—may well be acne's best friend. (More on the testosterone connection in a moment.)

Choose the Right Carbs

It's not just a high-carb diet that's responsible for the surge in insulin and its resulting effect on acne. The Kitavan Islanders ate a diet of almost 70 percent carbohydrates—but they never saw a Twinkie or a processed breakfast cereal. Their carbs came from tubers, fruits, and vegetables, which are considered a low-glycemic, or low-sugar, diet.

Although no one has investigated this directly, factory-farmed meat and chicken contain hormones and hormone-like compounds that can affect the body's hormonal balance and could certainly be part of the problem. Meat eaten in the native cultures where acne is virtually absent comes from wild game and pasture-fed (grass-fed) animals, not from factory farms where cows are routinely given large doses of hormones.

One study in the Journal of the *American Academy of Dermatology* investigated the relationship between diet and teenage acne and found a significant positive association between acne and milk (skim and whole). The researchers hypothesized that the association may be because of the "presence of hormones and bioactive molecules in milk."

Although no one is claiming that diet is the only cause of acne, no responsible nutritionist or health practitioner should deny the overwhelming evidence that a bad diet makes matters much worse. There are probably genetic factors that make one susceptible to excess keratin and sebum production and to the inflammation and infection that can contribute to acne. But eating in a way that produces excessive amounts of hormones that do the same thing may "turn on" those genes; eating a natural, traditional diet lower in sugar and processed foods does not.

Selling Health to Your Teens

Acne is also promoted by a diet low in the antioxidants found in abundance in vegetables and fruits. "Acne may be the best angle you will ever use to sell a healthy diet to your teenage children," says McDougall. "After all, millions of people living in Papua New Guinea, Paraguay, and rural Africa and Asia who eat a plant-based diet are acne-free throughout their lives—so why can't you also be acne-free if you behave like they do?"

A diet rich in plant foods provides huge amounts of antioxidants and natural anti-inflammatory agents. Whole foods are also high in fiber and low in sugar, and do not raise insulin to any levels that are likely to be problematic. Research going back to 1977 suggested that patients with acne may not metabolize sugar very well. Back in 1959, researchers writing in the Journal of the Canadian Medical Association went so far as to refer to acne as "skin diabetes." It appears they were on to something.

The Hormonal Connection

One of the main factors that drives the overproduction of either sebum or keratin is hormones. According to Michael Murray, N.D., acne is considered a "male hormone dependent condition" because the male hormone testosterone fuels the growth of keratin and causes the sebaceous glands to enlarge and

Natural Prescription for Acne

Paleo Diet: No grains, dairy, beans, or soy; high in protein (fish, grass-fed meats), vegetables, fruits (especially berries), nuts, and omega fats

May also be helpful: Saw palmetto 320 mg daily

overproduce sebum. (Don't forget—females also have testosterone, just not as much as we guys.) But it's not just the amount of testosterone you have that causes the problem. It's how your body metabolizes it.

Testosterone converts in the body to a nasty little compound called DHT—dihydrotestosterone—which stimulates the sebaceous glands to produce even higher levels of sebum. To complicate things further, a high glycemic diet accelerates the conversion of testosterone to DHT, one reason the low-sugar paleo diet works so well

When eating meat, grass-fed, hormone-free choices are less likely to contribute to the problem of acne because they don't add hormones to the diet. According to Robert Ivker, D.O., a diet of 45 percent protein appears to restrict the conversion of testosterone to DHT. My guess is simply reducing sugar and processed carbs—even if they weren't replaced with protein—would accomplish the same thing. The take-away message is that the processed foods that are rampant in the Western diet create a hormonal situation that is likely to seriously aggravate acne or even, in some cases, actually cause it.

Enter Saw Palmetto

Saw palmetto is an herb with a documented ability to prevent some of that conversion of testosterone to DHT. The question is, what role exactly does DHT play in acne? How much of hormone-driven acne is due to testosterone and how much is due to its metabolite DHT (which I like to call "son of testosterone") no one is quite sure. But it's very possible that DHT plays a substantial role, and if so, limiting the conversion of testosterone to DHT—which saw palmetto can clearly do—would be a boon for acne sufferers.

Fried, of my "go-to" guys for skin problems, explains it this way: "There are people who, through God, bad luck, or genes, are just susceptible to the effects of testosterone and DHT. The cells that line the hair follicle over-respond to this hormonal stimulation."

When this happens, the oil glands produce too much oil, which in turn clogs the follicles and creates a welcome environment for bacteria. "The immune system mounts an attack against that bacteria, which leads to inflammation, which is why a pimple can turn into a nasty, red cyst that can scar both physically and emotionally," Fried says. The theory—and it remains a theory—is that by downsizing the conversion of testosterone to DHT, saw palmetto can make a big difference.

Opinion is divided on saw palmetto as a natural cure for acne. Though as of this writing there aren't any solid research studies on acne and saw palmetto, there is a lot of anecdotal evidence from a growing number of people who've had good luck with it. It makes good common sense that it might be a terrific adjunct to the Paleolithic diet in a natural prescription for acne.

Aging Complications
Feel Young Again with this Combo Cure

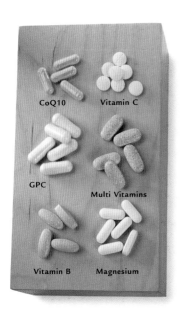

CoQ10   Vitamin C

GPC

Multi Vitamins

Vitamin B   Magnesium

IF YOU'RE A BABY BOOMER, at some point in your life you've undoubtedly heard yourself say the following words: "Senior moment!" And if you aren't a baby boomer, chances are you still know what your boomer friends mean when they say them. (If you don't, let me translate from boomer-ese. A "senior moment" means "I can't remember where I put my keys. Oh my God, is this the beginning of Alzheimer's?") Well, the good news is ... not necessarily. Not necessarily because some degree of memory loss—or what's clinically called cognitive decline—is expected as we grow older. It happens to many people, if not to everyone.

But there's good news. First, some amount of memory loss or cognitive decline doesn't necessarily translate to any meaningful impairment of your brain power or ability to function. Second, cognitive impairment doesn't always progress to Alzheimer's. And third, there are things you can do right now to protect your brain.

"The brain is like every other organ in the body, only more so. It's more delicate, more metabolically active, more easily damaged, requires more energy, and is in more need of serious nutritional and lifestyle support if it's to stay fit longer," says brain surgeon Larry McCleary, M.D., author of *The Brain Trust Program*.

The Cost of Aging

As of 2006, the youngest members of the group of more than 78 million people in the United States known as baby boomers will have passed their fortieth birthday. The older members of the group, which include George W. Bush and Bill Clinton (and me), turned sixty in this same year.

About 30 million of us will suffer some form of dementia, according to *New York Times* columnist David Brooks. A somewhat greater degree of decline, clinically known as mild cognitive impairment or MCI, will affect 10 percent of the over-65 population—about 15 percent of that group will go on to develop full-blown Alzheimer's. There are now more than five million people in the United States living with Alzheimer's, estimates the Alzheimer's Association. Someone develops Alzheimer's every seventy-two seconds, and, for what it's worth, the direct and indirect financial cost of Alzheimer's and other dementias have a price tag of more than $148 billion a year.

I'm sure I don't need to tell you that Alzheimer's and dementia are no laughing matters. Nor is the overall health of your brain. It's a major concern of many people in this country, particularly baby boomers or those of us who have had to care for aging parents with some form of dementia. It's not fun— not for them, not for us, and it's a fate every one of us would do anything to avoid. I can't promise you that the supplements in this combo cure will prevent Alzheimer's. But I can promise you that every one of them—separately or in combination—has been shown to produce improvements in mild cognitive impairment and/or in full-blown Alzheimer's.

(Brain) Size May Not Matter

You're born with roughly 100 billion neurons (brain cells), and the brain increases its mass about threefold until you reach your early twenties. (Which is why my friend Janet, when exasperated, frequently says to her teenage daughter, Molly, "I'll have this conversation with you in ten years when your brain is finished developing!")

The rate at which neurons die off is very individual, and, contrary to conventional wisdom, you continue to grow new ones all your life—it's just that the rate of growth slows down, while the rate of dying continues, leaving you with a somewhat smaller brain. By the age of eighty, your brain is about 10 percent smaller than it was when you were a quick-witted smart alec at age twenty. (Part of this is due to neurons shrinking as well as dying.)

But the good news is that brain size may not matter that much. While you lose neurons, your brilliantly resilient brain is able to continue to form new neural connections and pathways, meaning that the loss in size can easily be compensated by an increase in versatility and new learning. Your functional capacity needn't be deeply affected at all. That, of course, assumes you keep your brain healthy so it can maintain its ability to "retrain" itself, and continue to function sharply until the day you die. And you do that in three ways—with the foods you eat, the lifestyle choices you make, and the supplements you take.

Basic Brain Nutrition 101

Back in 2003, reports from the Chicago Health and Aging Project started documenting the powerful effects that nutrients can have on cognitive decline and Alzheimer's disease. The project was a study of common chronic health problems of older persons, and especially risk factors for Alzheimer's disease. These studies were conducted in a biracial neighborhood on the south side of Chicago. The researchers looked at more than 3,000 participants over the age of sixty-five and with a racial mix of 60 percent African American and 40 percent white. The simple executive summary of what they found is this: Nutrient deficiencies can increase the rate of cognitive decline. And adopting a few simple healthy eating habits—like including fish and vegetables in your regular diet—can slow down cognitive decline by the equivalent of up to nineteen years. Pretty impressive for a non-drug intervention, especially because that same dietary strategy (fish and vegetables) has been shown to reduce heart disease as well.

Food aside, certain nutrients continue to be mentioned, studied, and verified on the subject of preserving brain power. Used in combination, they are a powerhouse for mental protection.

Acetyl-L-Carnitine: The Memory Keeper

The mitochondria are tiny, two-membraned structures in the cytoplasm of the cell that are known as the cells' power source—they're little energy production factories where most of the chemical energy needed for life is generated. When your mitochondria are in trouble, so are you. The term for that—mitochondrial dysfunction—contributes to all sorts of human pathologies from neurodegenerative disease to stroke, heart attack, and diabetes. Neurosurgeon Russell Baylock, M.D., says acetyl-L-carnitine improves the function of the mitochondria, "returning them to the way they were when you were twenty."

Sign me up!

Acetyl-L-carnitine is a kind of supercharged version of carnitine that has a particularly positive effect in the brain. Carnitine acts as a shuttle, transporting fatty acids into the mitochondria where they can be "burned" for energy—one reason it's so important for the heart. Neurologist David Perlmutter, M.D., author of *The Better Brain Book*, describes acetyl-L-carnitine as a "neuronal energizer."

He also points out that it helps remove waste products from the mitochondria energy production factory, enabling them to be eliminated from the body.

"This is a very important job," he says. "If toxins are not removed from mitochondria, they can damage the mitochondria, which will slow down energy production even more."

Several clinical trials have suggested that acetyl-L-carnitine may delay the onset of age-related cognitive decline and improve overall cognitive function in the elderly. It also protects the brain from damage resulting from poor circulation and helps repair injured nerve cells. After three months using recommended doses of acetyl-L-carnitine, there is marked improvement in general cognitive function. One study found that a dose of 1,500 mg of acetyl-L-carnitine taken once a day for ninety days substantially improved reactions to stress, memory function, and mood.

Acetyl-L-carnitine helps the brain form acetylcholine, a neurotransmitter needed for memory and thinking. A number of studies have demonstrated positive effects of acetyl-L-carnitine supplementation in Alzheimer's patients, especially with regard to tasks that involve concentration and attention. One study done in 1991 and published in *Neurology* divided 130 Alzheimer's patients into two groups. One was treated with acetyl-L-carnitine while the other received a placebo. In thirteen of the fourteen outcome measures (including long-term verbal memory, selective attention, and logical intelligence), the acetyl-L-carnitine group had better scores. Those patients who had "good treatment compliance"—meaning they actually listened to the doctor and took their supplements on a regular basis—showed even greater benefit. More recent studies continue to show positive effects, but younger patients seem to benefit even more.

Perlmutter believes that carnitine is one of the few substances that can help slow down the progression of Alzheimer's, pointing out that people with Alzheimer's disease have "strikingly low levels of carnitine." According to the *Physician's Desk Reference*, preliminary evidence shows that acetyl-L-carnitine can slow mental decline in the elderly who are not afflicted with dementia. Perlmutter suggests that "supplementing with this vital amino acid in midlife, when levels begin to decline, may help prevent this brain degenerative disease in the first place."

Membranes Matter

Phosphatidylserine (PS) is a member of a class of biochemicals called phospholipids. It's a naturally occurring nutrient that's found in the cell membranes, but it's most concentrated in the brain. As neurologist Jay Lombard,

M.D., author of *The Brain Wellness Plan* says, "The first step in treating patients with Alzheimer's disease is to rebuild defective membranes."

Membranes matter.

PS has been available as a supplement for decades and has been shown in well-documented studies to restore brain function. It helps improve learning and name recall, concentration, face recognition, the ability to remember telephone numbers, and the ability to find misplaced objects. One of its primary functions is to regulate the release of various neurotransmitters.

"Our brain health depends on ... phosphatidylserine for a number of important metabolic effects," Lombard says, "including making it possible for nutrients to move freely in and out of neurons."

Steven Bratman, M.D., author of The Natural Health Encyclopedia, a database on herbs and supplements that many hospitals use, says that "... it is not a great leap to suspect that [PS might be] useful for much less severe problems with memory and mental function, such as those that seem to occur in nearly all of us who are older than forty." And my good friend, biochemist and nutritional supplement expert Parris Kidd, writes: "The findings from ... clinical trial(s) are unequivocal: dietary supplementation with PS can alleviate, ameliorate, and sometimes reverse age-related decline of memory, learning, concentration, word skills, and mood."

The Miracle Anti-Aging Nutrient for Your Brain

Glycerophosphocholine (GPC) is a supplement that has been extensively researched for its effect on mental performance, attention, concentration,

Natural Prescription for Aging Complications

Phosphatidylserine: 100 to 300 mg

Acetyl-L-carnitine: Start with 250 mg per day and increase up to 4,000 mg per day in divided doses

GPC: 300 to 1,200 mg in the morning

Alpha lipoic acid: 100 mg

Omega-3 fatty acids (either in capsules or liquid fish oil): 1,000 to 3,000 mg

B-complex vitamin: Include extra B12 (1,000 mcg may be best for older people)

CoQ10: 100 mg

Vitamin C: 1 to 2 g

Multiple vitamin and/or antioxidant formula: 1 per day or as directed

Magnesium: 800 IU

Diet: Increase vegetables (especially spinach), fish, and berries (especially blueberries); Drink green tea (two cups a day or more)

Exercise: Mild to moderate exercise at least three days a week

OPTIONAL:

Standardized ginkgo extract: 40 mg, three times a day (total 120 mg)

You can also take 60 mg, twice a day, or double up with 120 mg, twice a day

Vinpocentine: 10 mg, three times a day

Huperzine A: 60 to 200 mcg

Vitamin E (mixed tocopherols): 1,000 to 2,000 IU daily

Note: The above dosages are daily and in pill or capsule form, unless otherwise noted.

and memory formation. Like PS, it's a member of the class of biochemicals known as phospholipids, which are important in making healthy cell membranes. GPC is found in abundant quantities in mother's milk, which ought to tell us something about its importance in human life. There are only tiny amounts in food, so to get the full therapeutic value of this wonderful substance, supplements are the way to go.

A large body of scientific research has demonstrated GPC's importance for the brain. "I continue to be fascinated by GPC's capacities to salvage function in the damaged brain, to sharpen mental performance even in people who are healthy, and to give new vitality to the aging brain," Kidd says.

I'll tell you one of many examples that demonstrate the scientific validation of this remarkable nutrient. One set of trials involved a fascinating phenomenon called scopolamine amnesia. It seems that if you administer a chemical called scopolamine (by injection or by mouth) to people, they will very quickly experience near-total amnesia. They just forget everything. It's remarkable—all information skills, including memory, attention, and learning, just seem to disappear. The chemical is harmless, the effect is only temporary, and it wears off in a few hours, but it allows researchers to do all sorts of clever studies.

In two of these studies, researchers first gave healthy young volunteers GPC or a placebo over the course of a week to ten days. Then they gave them the scopamine injection and watched them carefully for the next six hours. They wanted to determine the degree to which GPC could protect their minds against the (inevitable) amnesia brought on by the drug.

The researchers had the subjects perform a test called free recall (twenty words are read aloud three times and subjects have two minutes to write down as many as they can remember), and a test of attention called the cancellation test (subjects are given a matrix of 1,200 randomly generated numbers and told to find three that are identified as "targets" and eliminate them from the matrix within three minutes).

The results were pretty amazing. In the free recall test, the GPC held off the amnesia all the way through the six-hour trial. In the cancellation test, it held off the amnesia for three hours (a partial but very real effect on attention). The researchers concluded that GPC protected the brain's attention and memory capacity. Even more interestingly, the GPC group scored higher in a baseline test of word recall—given to all subjects before they were given the scopolamine, meaning the seven to ten days of treatment with GPC had had a positive effect on their brains even before the experiment began!

Kidd sums it up best when he says, "Along with its sister phospholipid PS, GPC has a proven track record against age-related decline and other brain damage. These are the two most clinically proven brain nutrients, and both are widely needed, especially since there are no pharmaceuticals available that provide lasting benefit against cognitive decline." If you use this supplement, take it in the morning, as it's possible that taking it late in the day may keep you up well after you're ready for bed.

Other Cognitive Defenders

Alpha lipoic acid, first gained attention as a potential brain nutrient through the work of one of the most respected researchers in nutrition and biochemistry, Bruce Ames, Ph.D. Ames, a professor of the graduate school division of biochemistry and molecular biology at the University of California, performed a series of experiments in which he gave aging rats a combination of acetyl-L-carnitine and lipoic acid. Animals taking the mix performed better on memory tests and also showed general signs of vitality.

"With these two supplements together, these old rats got up and did the Macarena," Ames says. "The brain looks better, they are full of energy—everything we looked at looks more like a young animal." Indeed, analysis of the rats' brain tissue showed that they had less damage to the mitochondria—the power centers of the cells—and less oxidative damage to the memory center of the brain (the hippocampus).

Some researchers—notably neurologist Perlmutter—suggest that alpha lipoic acid's usefulness as a brain nutrient may be because of its powerful effect as an antioxidant, including its ability to significantly boost what Perlmutter considers the brain's most important antioxidant, glutathione. As an antioxidant, alpha lipoic acid helps protect against devastating damage from rogue molecules called free radicals. "If your brain is being devoured by free radicals, you will not be able to think clearly, stay focused, or retrieve information when you need it," he says.

But don't stop there!

Vinpocentine is a chemical substance synthesized from vincamine, a natural constituent found in the leaves of a plant in the periwinkle family (Vinca minor). While it's not a superstar nutrient in the cognitive arsenal, it does seem to have some effect. In one multicenter, double-blind, placebo-controlled sixteen-week study, patients with "mild to moderate" cognitive impairment problems were treated with vinpocetine. They were then tested on cognitive performance tests and on measures of "global improvement." Their results were compared with the results of a similar group that received placebo, and those treated with vinpocentine did significantly better. Another study tested vinpocentine against a placebo in elderly patients with cerebrovascular (circulation in the brain) and central nervous system degenerative disorders, and similarly good results were found. Vinpocentine so far has not been shown to be helpful with Alzheimer's, but it may improve blood flow in the brain.

Then there's **vitamin B12**, which is essential for the proper functioning of the brain. B12 plays an important role in creating and maintaining the protective coating around neurons, called the myelin sheath. Because B12 is necessary for proper nerve conduction, if and when you have less of it, the nerve impulses or messages are less effective at getting to their destinations, so B12 is essential for the proper functioning of the brain. A deficiency of B12 may lead to mental disorders including confusion, depression, memory loss, and impaired coordination.

Vitamin B12 is also protective against the toxic buildup of another substance called homocysteine. In an article in the prestigious *New England Journal of Medicine*, researchers from the department of neurology at Boston University School of Medicine found that a high level of homocysteine in the blood "is a strong, independent risk factor for the development of dementia and Alzheimer's disease." Homocysteine levels are easily brought back down by vitamin B12, vitamin B6, and folic acid. It is quite common for the elderly to be deficient in B12. In one study reported in *The Archives of Internal Medicine* in 2006, researchers gave subjects B12 injections once per day for a week, then weekly for a month, then monthly thereafter for six to twelve months. "Striking improvements" in cognitive function and anemia were noted.

Vitamin B12 doesn't work alone, however. Having adequate amounts of all the B vitamins, especially folic acid and vitamin B6, is also critical for protection against homocysteine and cognitive decline. All work together nicely to reduce homocysteine levels and protect against anemias as well as mental disorders.

The trio of vitamin B6, vitamin B12, and folic acid is the best remedy for eliminating the risk factor of homocysteine.

Ginkgo for Memory Enhancement

If you're healthy, young, and have no particular health issues or memory problems, taking ginkgo isn't going to help you ace an exam that you would have otherwise failed, or suddenly start remembering what you had for breakfast four days ago. But that doesn't mean ginkgo doesn't have important effects on the brain and other aspects of your health. It does.

The overwhelming majority of research studies have demonstrated that ginkgo supplementation has a positive effect on cognition. There have been numerous double-blind, placebo-controlled studies that show ginkgo extract is effective in reducing either the progress of dementia or the severity of its symptoms. The results are not always dramatic, but they are significant.

A number of studies have shown that ginkgo modestly improves both memory and the speed of cognitive functioning, as well as the symptoms of Alzheimer's and vascular or mixed dementia. Some studies even show that ginkgo leaf extract can stabilize or improve some measures of cognitive and social functioning in patients with multiple types of dementia. In Germany, physicians are so sure of ginkgo's benefits that it's hard to get them to perform scientific studies of the herb.

"To them, it is unethical to give a placebo to people with Alzheimer's when they could be taking ginkgo instead and have additional months of useful life ahead", says Bratman. Other studies that examined the effects of ginkgo on men and women who didn't suffer from any mental impairment have also demonstrated improvements in mental functioning. "The scientific record for ginkgo is extensive and impressive," Bratman says.

Ginkgo is by far the most widely prescribed herb in Germany, reaching more than $200 million in sales (for 1996). There are at least two proprietary ginkgo medicines (Tebonin and Rokan) on the market in Germany.

The most studied form of ginkgo biloba is an extract called EGB 761. Try to find a brand that has been standardized for that extract. (One such brand in the United States is Ginkgold by Nature's Way.) According to the Herb Research Foundation, look for extracts that have been standardized for 24 percent ginkgo flavone glycosides. Some researchers suggest that the combination of ginkgo and Panax ginseng might be even more effective than either used alone. Give ginkgo at least a twelve-week trial, the length of time usedin many studies.

The Role of Acetylcholine

Although the complete story of what causes what in Alzheimer's may remain unclear for a while, many scientists suspect that at least part of the picture has to do with an important chemical called acetylcholine. Deficiencies in acetylcholine can affect memory and thinking, and researchers suspect that at the very least, this is a contributing factor in dementia, and possibly even ordinary memory loss.

Acetylcholine is what's called a neurotransmitter—a chemical produced in the brain that transmits information. Acetylcholine is absolutely essential for memory, attention, and thought. The cells that produce acetylcholine are among the first to die off in Alzheimer's disease. Parkinson's disease, dementia that results from multiple strokes, multiple sclerosis, and schizophrenia are all, like Alzheimer's, associated with lower levels of acetylcholine in the brain.

Acetylcholine is broken down in the brain by an enzyme called *acetylcholinesterase*. If you could somehow inhibit the action of this enzyme—making it perform its job less efficiently—you'd have more acetylcholine hanging around in the brain. Some Alzheimer's medicines—notably Aricept—work in just this way.

Huperzine Lends a Helping Hand

Enter huperzine A, a natural acetylcholinesterase inhibitor. By blocking the breakdown of acetylcholine it essentially increases the levels of acetylcholine hanging around your neurons. And while that doesn't "cure" Alzheimer's or address some of the other myriad issues in the Alzheimer's brain (like the plaques and tangles), it's still a very good thing indeed. Huperzine A has been shown to improve memory, thinking, and behavioral function in people with Alzheimer's disease, dementia caused by multiple strokes, and senile dementia.

Various types of huperzine A are available, and the natural form is about three times stronger and more potent than the synthetic kind. Doses of natural huperzine A used in the studies ranges from 60 to 200 mcg daily. *The Physicians' Desk Reference* suggests that you use it with a physician's recommendation and monitoring.

The Fountain of Youth

Genetic makeup is partly responsible for determining the rate at which people lose cognitive function and whether they will develop dementia, but lifestyle choices play a huge role as well. So does diet.

Just ask James Joseph. Joseph, Ph.D., a scientist at the Laboratory of Neuroscience at the U.S. Department of Agriculture's Human Nutrition Research Center on Aging at Tufts University, has a special interest in what we should eat if we want to keep our marbles intact as we grow older. In Joseph's lab, he's got something he calls the rat Olympics. He tests motor function and memory function with mazes and assorted tests for muscle strength and coordination. Around middle age, rats start showing the same kinds of decline in performance that humans do. But Joseph's studies show that when you feed lab animals extracts of blueberries, wonderful things start happening—or, more accurately, bad things don't happen.

Such as mental deterioration.

Rats that chow down on blueberries in the Joseph lab act like they've found the Rat Fountain of Youth. Blueberries actually help neurons in the brain communicate with one another more effectively.

"Old neurons are kind of like old married couples," Joseph says. "They don't talk to each other so much anymore." Memory goes down and the "processing" necessary for coordination and balance tends to decline. The technical term for this communication is signaling, and special compounds in blueberries called polyphenols actually "turn on" the signals. "Not only can you get one neuron to talk to another more efficiently, but you can actually enable the brain to grow new neurons," Joseph explains in an interview. "Call the blueberry the brain berry."

While blueberries have emerged as a superfood for the brain, they're not the only food that has an effect. Researchers writing in the *Journal of Neuroscience* reported rats that consumed an extract of blueberries, strawberries, and spinach every day showed improvements in short-term memory.

And let's not forget the value of fish and fish oil. Inflammation is a big component of every degenerative disease, including Alzheimer's, and fish oil is one of the most anti-inflammatory substances on the planet. Your grandma was right when she told you fish was brain food. About 60 percent of your brain is fat, and most of that is an omega-3 fatty acid known as docosahexaenoic acid or DHA. Where is it found, you ask? In fish. I consider omega-3s one of the most protective supplements you can take for many reasons, not the least of which that they go a long way toward protecting your brain.

Niacin intake from foods has also been shown to be inversely associated with Alzheimer's disease. Higher intake of niacin from food has been shown in some research to be associated with a slower annual rate of cognitive decline. Foods like eggs, liver, fish, and broccoli are great sources. Bottom line: Eat your fruits and vegetables, but don't forget your fats and protein.

The Power of the Crossword Puzzle

Much has been written about mental aerobics, brain teasers, and other ways of keeping your brain young. Obviously all that good press for mental gymnastics has had an impact (what other possible reason could there be for the popularity of Sudoku?).

Research at the National Institutes of Health showed that seniors who practiced certain thinking skills maintained their ability to perform those skills better than those who didn't practice them. I've often believed one of the reasons symphonic conductors live so long and conduct well into their seventies and eighties and beyond is because they're constantly studying new scores. They're also throwing their arms around a lot—and don't think for a minute that mild aerobic exercise doesn't have an effect on your brain. It does. Women who exercise regularly have a 20 percent risk decrease for cognitive impairment. Additionally, physical activity can improve reaction time, memory span, and overall well-being. One study reports that going for walks may be enough to stem the age-related decline in physical reaction time.

Recent research shows that regular exercise can not only increase the ability of the brain to function, but it can actually increase its size. Arthur Kramer, Ph.D., professor of neuroscience and psychology and director of the biomedical imaging center at the University of Illinois, and his colleagues demonstrated this in an intriguing study. They put a group of sixty volunteers in an MRI machine, which can pinpoint changes and abnormalities in body tissues.

"These folks were basically couch potatoes," Kramer told me, "healthy but sedentary, and ranging in age from sixty to eighty." The researchers then divided

Avoid the Number-One Brain Shrinker

I've written elsewhere about the effect of stress hormones on weight. Executive summary: Stress makes you fat. And now I'm going to give you more bad news: It also shrinks your brain.

No kidding.

An important structure in the brain essential to memory called the hippocampus actually shrinks as a result of stress. The total number of cells decreases, and if that weren't bad enough, the existing cells shrink. (The hippocampus is also one of the first regions to suffer damage in Alzheimer's disease.) A ton of research has validated this shrinkage, and this chapter is long enough as it is, so I'm going to give you the bottom line: If you don't handle your stress, bad things will happen.

Stress aggravates virtually every disease and condition we've talked about in this book, and in some cases, it makes the difference between really bad symptoms and mild ones you can easily live with. The effect of chronic levels of stress hormones on the brain is incalculable. If you think you can't afford to take the time to do some stress-reducing activities, rethink that.

You can't afford not to.

Ways to reduce stress are as easy to find as your own bathroom. A soak in a warm bath works wonders, especially when you add some Epsom salts (loaded with relaxing magnesium). Ditto lying in bed by candlelight reading a book that doesn't have anything to do with work. Making love works great, plus it raises both your serotonin and the bonding hormone oxytocin. Try spending time with an animal. Or in the sunshine. (Better yet—spend time with an animal in the sunshine!) Meditation is probably the most reliable and proven way to bring down stress hormones, but if that's not your cup of tea try some simple breathing exercises. (There's a reason they tell you to take a deep breath when you're boiling mad—deep breathing and stress are incompatible).

Whatever you choose, do something.

Ultimately the health of your brain depends on it.

them into two groups. One group went into an aerobics program, the other into a "toning and stretching" program.

"The aerobics group started at fifteen minutes a day, at a pretty slow pace," Kramer says, "but after two months they were up to forty-five to sixty minutes, three days a week." This continued for six months, after which the subjects went back into the MRI machine, and the researchers examined their gray and white matter. (The gray matter of the brain is composed of neurons or computational units, while the white matter is the axons, or interconnections—"telephone wires between the neurons," says Kramer.)

Both the gray matter and the white matter showed increased volume, showing that exercise can literally build up your brain. And the best part is that it doesn't take much. A pretty moderate level can do the trick, in this case just walking forty-five to sixty minutes, three times a week.

And even if you don't much care about the physical size of your brain, exercise has also been shown to reduce the risk of Alzheimer's disease and other forms of dementia. One theory is that it does so by increasing blood flow to the brain. A study in *the Archives of Internal Medicine* evaluated the cognitive functioning of seniors over the age of sixty-five for almost six years and found that the less they exercised, the quicker the rate of cognitive decline and the higher the risk for dementia, including Alzheimer's disease. In a sobering finding, those who didn't exercise were three times more likely to develop dementia.

Green Tea Cuts Risk of Cognitive Impairment

One easy thing you can do right now to protect your brain is to drink green tea on a daily basis. A 2006 study showed that elderly Japanese people who consumed more than two cups of green tea a day had a 50 percent lower chance of having cognitive impairment compared to those who drank fewer than two cups a day, (or who consumed other tested beverages). Researchers suspect this may be due to the effect of an important plant compound called EGCG (epigallocatechin gallate), which has also been found to have metabolism-boosting and anti-cancer properties as well.

Allergies, Seasonal and Food-Related

Consider This Combo Cure for Relief—and Answers

THERE ARE THREE THINGS you need to know about allergies. One: They come in two basic flavors—food allergies and seasonal (airborne) allergies. Two: Seasonal allergies can be made worse by problem foods. Three: "Real" food allergies are pretty rare; annoying and debilitating "food reactions" are common. (Many people use the word "allergy" to describe what is actually a food sensitivity.) No matter which you suffer with, you'll find something in this chapter of interest.

Candied Citrus Peel

Quercetin

Vitamin C

Stinging Nettles

Seasonal Allergies

Seasonal allergies are characterized by inflammation of the mucous membranes in the nasal passages. Airborne pollens from grasses, flowers, weeds, trees, or ragweed are the culprits, so allergy season officially begins whenever trees and grasses start to pollinate in your area of the country.

Why do these innocuous little molecules cause so much suffering in the first place? Well, these airborne little buggers, which can be pollens or even chemicals, get absorbed through the lungs or skin into the blood and cause the white blood cells of allergy-prone folks to produce a ton of an antibody known as IgE (immunoglobulin E). This is the same immunoglobulin that's triggered in a classic food allergy, only this time it's triggered by something you breathe rather than eat. The offending molecules then travel through the bloodstream and hit cells called mast cells, which are major storage sites for histamine. Once the mast cell takes a hit from the IgE antibody, it begins "leaking" histamine all over the place, producing the familiar and annoying symptoms everyone who suffers from seasonal allergies knows all too well.

Conventional medicine doesn't have a lot to offer. Antihistamines like Benadryl and Tavist D can help, but they can cause drowsiness. Nasal decongestants can help, but they're also not without possible side effects (restlessness, irritability, and insomnia are among the most common). And while most of these are probably safe, I can't help remembering that one "safe" nasal decongestant—*phenylpropanolamine*—was pulled off the market a few years ago after it was found to be linked to an increased risk of hemorrhagic stroke in women aged 18 to 49. Wouldn't it be great if there were some powerful natural treatment for seasonal allergies?

Well, there is. And it's a bioflavonoid called *quercetin*. Combined with a few other things (including the delicious Dr. Starbucks Fruit Peel, recipe below), it just might be your most powerful natural weapon against the annoying symptoms of seasonal allergies.

Quercetin to the Rescue

Quercetin is effective for allergies for the same reason it's effective for asthma—it's a powerful anti-inflammatory agent. It also has an "affinity" for mast cells, tending to stabilize their membranes and helping to prevent them from pouring out histamine in response to the IgE antibody.

Jaimison Starbuck, N.D., a naturopathic physician and past president of the American Association of Naturopathic Physicians, is a huge fan of quercetin. "It strengthens the capillaries in the upper respiratory tract to make them less reactive to the kind of inhalants that trigger allergic symptoms," she says.

Sometimes people with hay fever simply have very reactive mucous membranes, meaning they have a low threshold for irritation. These membranes may be slightly inflamed to begin with, or tend toward inflammation at the slightest irritation. "Quercetin tends to decrease inflammation, and it helps support the immune system at the same time," Starbuck told me. "I've had clients who just used quercetin alone and it makes a huge difference in their symptoms and suffering."

Fighting Food Allergies

Seasonal allergies are definitely aggravated by food allergies. Starbuck told me about an eight-year-old boy who was brought into her office by his mother,

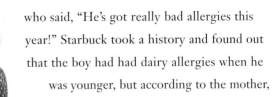

who said, "He's got really bad allergies this year!" Starbuck took a history and found out that the boy had had dairy allergies when he was younger, but according to the mother, "not anymore." "Just for fun, why don't you take him off dairy for a while?" Starbuck suggested. Can you guess what happened?

Wheat, dairy, corn, soy, or any of the other common foods that cause food sensitivities can aggravate a seasonal allergy and send it into overdrive. Remember, too, that dairy, wheat, and soy are all potentially mucus-producing foods. A nice, low-tech "elimination" diet might be just the ticket, at least during the allergy season. Take the offending foods out of the diet for a while and see whether your hay fever symptoms get better. Better yet, combine an elimination diet with the natural prescription for seasonal allergies and you might find you can throw your over-the-counter medications away, or at least reduce your use of them significantly.

But Which Foods Should I Eliminate?

There are a million tests for food allergies or "sensitivities," and everyone has their favorites—blood tests where they expose a little of your blood to ninety different foods and see what happens, saliva tests, you name it. All have their partisans and all have their detractors.

But there's a better way. It's low tech and—best of all—free. Plus it's likely to give you just as useful and meaningful a result as the most expensive of the "food sensitivity" tests.

It's called the *rotation*, or *elimination* diet. And it's by far one of the best and most reliable methods for identifying foods that might cause you a variety of health problems.

WORTH KNOWING

Because this is detective work, it would be wise to keep a food journal while you begin your program. After all, Holmes and Watson always used one to crack their crimes. This is no different. You must find the culprits. Writing down how you feel after you eat and paying attention to any symptoms will give you clues and lead you to the cause.

I'm not suggesting you try the rotation diet with foods that have triggered serious, potentially life-threatening reactions. (If you've gone into anaphylactic shock when eating peanuts, don't eat peanuts. Period.) We're talking here about foods that produce annoying, vague, hard-to-pin-down symptoms that you may not even have suspected as being food related. For goodness' sake, do not try this with any foods that have triggered a life-threatening response in the past. I'm sure you know this, but it's worth mentioning anyway.

The Rotation Diet Explained

A rotation diet simply means that you rotate the foods that you eat every four to five days, or longer, depending on how you react to each one. In the classic version, you first eliminate the common offenders—sugar, wheat, and dairy—for thirty days. (That little trio of usual suspects is responsible for more unexplained symptoms than you can possibly imagine.)

Then, at the start of the second month, you would, for instance, eat wheat on Day 1. You would not be able to eat any kind of wheat again until Day 5 or 6. You may find that you can eat some of the foods that are on rotation every fourth day with no problems, but that others must be rotated at longer intervals for you to tolerate them. Eating the allergenic foods on a rotated basis reduces your exposure to them and also reduces your sensitivity to them so that you are better able to tolerate them. The general thinking is that after four or five days you have completely excreted the food from your body, so there is no risk of a buildup of allergenic toxins.

Allan D. Lieberman, M.D., director at the Center for Occupational and Environmental Medicine in South Carolina, is one of many practitioners who believe we should all think about rotating our foods. Rotation not only helps to reveal hidden food allergies and prevent new allergies from developing, but by allowing us to identify offending foods—and then putting a temporary "off limits" sign on them—we give our immune systems a needed break, Lieberman says. Hidden food allergies can cause digestive problems that will send the immune system on an all-out alert, creating inflammation and a host of other symptoms. By removing the problem

Natural Prescription for Allergies, Seasonal and Food-Related

Try a rotation or elimination diet. Start by eliminating grains (or at the very least wheat) and dairy.

Natural Prescription for Seasonal Allergies

Quercetin: 300 mg, three times a day (When symptoms are under control, you can go down to 500 to 1,000 mg once a day.)

Stinging nettles (optional): 600 mg, freeze-dried extract

Vitamin C: 1,000 to 2,000 mg

Dr. Starbuck's candied fruit peels: Several times a day. Recipe: Using organic produce, wash and peel an orange, a grapefruit, and a lemon. Cut the peels into bite-size pieces (you're welcome to eat the fruit, but it's not part of this concoction). Mix water and organic honey together in a 50-50 mix based on the amount you want to make. Bring the mix to a simmer, but don't boil it because boiling will kill the bioactive bioflavonoids in the peels. Add the peels and simmer until they are soft and coated with the honey mix. Cool in the fridge and eat like candy.

foods the immune system is better able to heal and stay strong. Best of all, rotation diets allow us to eventually eat the foods we love—just less of them. And less frequently.

Most people use rotation diets as a first plan of attack when they suspect a food allergy, but a rotation diet can also be a good all-around starting point for other symptoms that just can't be explained any other way: fatigue, achy joints, eczema, irritable bowel, or a depressed immune function. If you've already been diagnosed with certain food allergies or sensitivities, a rotation is the very best place to start.

The European Congress of Allergology and Clinical Immunology (1999) conducted a study of 275 patients and found food connections to a wide variety of conditions including migraines, depression, hypertension, angina, irritable bowel syndrome (IBS), and eczema. For instance, people with IBS showed "remarkable" improvement with the elimination of pineapple, citrus, cantaloupe, bread, pork, and cheese (not necessarily all for the same patient!). In another study of fifty-seven patients with asthma, fruits were the most common triggers and—combined with milk, beef, lamb, pork, fish, and grain products—were by far the most common cause of food-related asthma symptoms.

Bottom line: The triggers are going to be different for different people, so you have to do your own science experiment with you as the subject. Take your health in your own hands and figure out what's really going on. When you identify the foods that cause your symptoms—or contribute to them—it's one of the most liberating experiences you can imagine. You may feel better than you have in years—even more so because you took charge of your own health.

Anxiety

Calm Your Nerves with Theanine

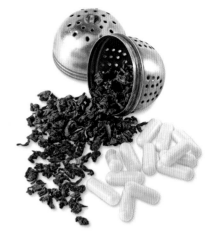

EVER WONDER WHY green-tea drinkers never seem to get the "hypers" that coffee drinkers get, even though the green tea is fully caffeinated?

The answer in all likelihood is a non-protein amino acid found in tea called *theanine*. Theanine is helpful in improving mood and increasing a sense of relaxation. In fact, it's used in Japan for just that purpose. The calming effect of theanine is probably the reason that drinking green tea—even with caffeine—doesn't produce nearly as jittery an experience as drinking coffee. If you want to relax, a theanine supplement might be just the thing for you.

Historically, theanine has been used for its ability to reduce anxiety and its overall calming effects. It is known to block the binding of *L-glutamic acid*— a neurotransmitter that "excites" or stimulates the brain—to its receptors. If you think of the little glutamic acid molecules as lamps and the receptors as wall outlets, theanine basically closes down some of those wall outlets so fewer lamps get plugged in and there's less bright light; the brain is then less "excited."

A 1999 study measured the brain activity of volunteers after an oral dose of 50 to 200 mg of L-theanine (also known as just *theanine*) and found that the supplement helped generate alpha brain waves, which are associated with relaxation. That may be another way that L-theanine helps promote relaxation. Theanine also seems to promote increased levels of gamma aminobutyric acid or GABA, an inhibitory neurotransmitter that also has significant calming effects in the brain. Some supplements actually combine theanine with GABA. (According to Ray Sahelian, M.D., GABA seems to work better when combined with other stress supplements, which explains why a theanine-GABA supplement like ZEN is one of the most popular supplements on my website, www.jonnybowden.com.)

I have a good friend who has one of the highest-pressure jobs in the United States—he's a CIA agent. As you can imagine, his wife has a bit of stress and anxiety in her daily life. (File that under "ya think?") He told me that theanine has been a lifesaver in their home. His wife says that a 200 mg theanine supplement takes the edge off anxiety, without making her the least bit drowsy. Maybe it can do the same for you.

Though B vitamins are often associated with energy, one in particular, B6, is necessary to make both GABA and the "relaxing" neurotransmitter, serotonin. Make sure you're getting all your B vitamins with a good B-complex, which will usually contain all the B6 you need. According to my friend Jacob Teitelbaum, M.D., low levels of vitamin B-12 have also been shown to be associated with anxiety.

Another member of the B family called *inositol* may also be helpful. Though it hasn't been studied specifically for anxiety or sleep, anecdotal evidence suggests that it's good for both. Research shows that it's helpful for treating panic disorders and possibly obsessive-compulsive disorder. I personally take about 6 grams in powdered form, mixed in a glass of water, before bed on nights when I'm feeling jittery. It definitely helps. (You can get the powdered form of inositol on my website, www.jonnybowden.com.)

Finally, don't forget magnesium. It's nature's muscle relaxant and can help with sleep and anxiety as well (think Epsom salts—the ultimate magnesium supplement!). Most people don't get enough of this important mineral, so a 400 to 800 mg daily dose certainly won't hurt and may help take the edge off.

Natural Prescription for Anxiety

Theanine: 200 mg

Also useful:

GABA: 200 to 500 mg (combined with
theanine in ZEN available at www.jonnybowden.com)

Inositol: 500 to 1,500 mg

Magnesium: 400 to 800 mg a day

Note: All dosages are daily dosages and in pill or capsule form unless otherwise noted.

Arthritis

Ease the Pain with Glucosamine and Chondroitin

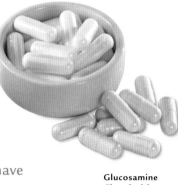

MSM

Glucosamine
Chondroitin
Sulfate

OSTEOARTHRITIS is one of the most common of the chronic health conditions. About two-thirds of all people older than sixty-five have physical signs of it that you can actually see on an x-ray, but many don't know they have it because they have no symptoms.

For others, the symptoms range from mildly annoying (a pain in the joint when it rains) to downright debilitating. After all, when cartilage in the joints wears down, eventually you're left with little or no shock absorbers—just bone rubbing on bone. That hurts. And over time, this rubbing will permanently damage the joint. Any joint can be affected; though it's very common in the knees, arthritis can also affect the hips, neck, lower spine, hands, and feet.

Talk to anyone knowledgeable about natural treatments for arthritis and joint pain, and one of the first things you're likely to hear about is glucosamine.

Interestingly, I was hearing about glucosamine from veterinarians long before the medical establishment decided to get on board with it. Vets tend to be way more open-minded about supplements than medical doctors; they simply use whatever works. And glucosamine works. It helps dogs—and people—with the pain, stiffness, and infirmity of arthritis. Remember, there are no placebo effects with dogs. They don't get better because they *think* they're supposed to—they either feel (and act) better or they don't.

And if their behavior is any indication, their joints seem to feel a lot better when they're given a hefty dose of glucosamine.

So do ours.

A Vital Building Block

Glucosamine is naturally synthesized in the human body and is a basic building block of connective tissue—like the cartilage in your knee, for example. Although we have an ample amount of the stuff when we're young, we lose some of it as we age, leading to the thinning of cartilage, which frequently progresses to osteoarthritis.

Glucosamine—and its partner chondroitin—can help.

Many studies have shown that glucosamine and/or chondroitin are beneficial in helping to repair damage to the joints caused by osteoarthritis (more on chondroitin in a minute). Though glucosamine can't bring cartilage back, it *can* prevent further loss as well as reduce symptoms of pain, swelling, and stiffness in the joints.

This is important, especially for postmenopausal women, who have a greater propensity toward osteoarthritis than men. In two independent, three-year, randomized, placebo-controlled studies, glucosamine sulfate was shown to slow the progression of osteoarthritis symptoms. After three years, post-menopausal participants in the groups given the glucosamine sulfate showed no joint space narrowing whatsoever, while those given a placebo did. Not only that, the glucosamine sulfate group showed a significant improvement in a standardized measure of pain called the WOMAC Index, while there was a trend for *worsening* of pain in the placebo group.

Let's face it: Joint pain is uncomfortable and frustrating, especially for those who are used to living an active life. For relief from the pain, many reach for remedies like the prescription drugs in the category known as COX-2 inhibitors (Celebrex and Vioxx are famous examples), or pain relievers such as acetaminophen (Tylenol) and nonsteroidal anti-inflammatory drugs (Aleve). These drugs do offer immediate relief, but they're hardly without problems (witness the class-action suits over Vioxx).

Keep in mind that none of these drugs (prescription or over-the-counter) addresses the underlying cause of the joint pain. Natural supplements like glucosamine not only help with pain—albeit a bit more slowly than drugs do—but unlike drugs, they have the potential to stop the progression of the condition that's causing it. Best of all, they do so without any serious side effects. And supplements like fish oil and shea nut oil (more on both in a moment) have significant anti-inflammatory properties. Inflammation *always* accompanies joint pain, so anything that reduces inflammation will help reduce the discomfort associated with arthritis.

The Role of Chondroitin

Chondroitin sulfate is another building block of connective tissue. It actually stimulates the cartilage cells (called chondrocytes), and therefore works beautifully when paired with glucosamine to speed the regeneration and recovery of bone tissues. While chondroitin taken alone doesn't seem to do very much, when taken together with glucosamine it offers significantly greater improvement of osteoarthritis than when either is used separately.

The Annual Scientific Meeting of the American College of Rheumatology in 2005 reported that the combination of glucosamine and chondroitin sulfate is at least as effective as the prescription drug celecoxib (brand name Celebrex) in treating pain caused by moderate to severe osteoarthritis of the knee. So for best results, use them together.

Glucosamine/chondroitin therapy requires patience: You may have to wait anywhere from eight to twelve weeks to see results. (The pain-relieving effects of omega-3s, however, are much more immediate.)

To increase the odds that you'll be among the many people who reap the benefits of this terrific natural combination, use them properly. There are different versions (called salts) of glucosamine, including glucosamine sulfate, glucosamine hydrochloride, and glucosamine hydroiodide.

Most studies have used glucosamine sulfate, so unless you're allergic to sulfates, that's probably your safest bet. The best studies used 1,500 mg of glucosamine sulfate a day, though I've heard some health practitioners swear by the idea of "loading up" with 3,000 mg a day for the first month and then dropping down to the recommended 1,500 mg. Some evidence suggests the dose has to be adjusted for obesity. Chondroitin seems to work well at around 800 to 1,500 mg daily.

Adding to the Arsenal

In addition to glucosamine sulfate and chondroitin sulfate, other nutrients have been shown to have benefits and may work synergistically with glucosamine and chondroitin.

WORTH KNOWING

In those patients who are obese, have peptic ulcers, or take diuretics, the effectiveness of glucosamine sulfate is reduced. So if this applies to you, work with a health-care provider to increase the doses shown on page 63.

Those who are allergic to sulfates may take glucosamine hydrochloride and not glucosamine sulfate, and they should avoid chondroitin sulfate. Glucosamine is derived from shrimp, oyster, and crab shells, and chondroitin is derived from cartilage of cows, pigs, and sharks. There is no synthetically made glucosamine on the market.

Glucosamine and chondroitin help regrow cartilage. However, if you have no cartilage left, these nutrients will not do artificial knees any good. They may help, though, with your other joints. The best option is to prevent the joint from getting to a stage of destruction by using nutrients that help keep cartilage tissue healthy. And to load up on anti-inflammatories like fish oil!

Methyl sulfonylmethane (MSM) is terrific for joint pain, largely because of its high sulfur content. (There's a reason people all over the world flock to hot sulfur baths for pain relief.) MSM blocks the transmission of impulses in nerve fibers that carry pain signals. Studies in laboratory animals whose diet included MSM showed less degenerative change of the articular joint compared to the control group. In the June 2004 journal *Clinical Drug Investigations*, scientists reported that glucosamine and MSM individually improved pain and swelling in arthritic joints; the combination of the two was more effective in reducing symptoms and improving the function of joints.

For Immediate Relief

In treating any inflammatory condition like arthritis, we never want to over-look the king of the natural anti-inflammatories, omega-3 fatty acids (fish oil). Fish oil works by reducing the number of inflammatory messenger molecules made by the body's immune system. The Arthritis Foundation recommends eating at least two fish meals a week—particularly fatty fish such as salmon, mackerel, and sardines. High-quality fish oil supplements are an excellent way to get the many health benefits of the omega-3 fatty acids.

I think the recommendation of the Arthritis Foundation is way too con-servative. I've seen hundreds of people get substantial relief from the pain and inflammation of arthritis (and other inflammatory conditions) by taking 2 to 3 grams of high-quality fish oil on a daily basis. I recommend Barlean's High Potency EPA-DHA (available on my website, www.jonnybowden.com). Whichever product you take, look at the label to see how much EPA and DHA it contains. If you can manage to take the liquid form, you'll be getting a wonderful dose just by taking one tablespoon a day—or even one to two teaspoons. Barlean's makes a fruit-flavored fish oil called Omega Swirl that tastes amazing and has no fishy aftertaste.

Another supplement that's been getting a lot of attention recently is shea nut oil. Shea nuts, found in Africa, can contain high levels of tripertenes, natural plant compounds that are highly anti-inflammatory. A recent study in *Phytotherapy Research* found that high-tripertene shea nut oil (available over the counter as "FlexNow" or, in a professional version as BSP, available on my website) found that those who took the supplement as directed experienced significant decreases in inflammation and cartilage breakdown.

Exercise for Arthritis

You may feel like exercise is out of the question if you have arthritis. Not so.

Moderate exercise can be your best friend—building strong muscles around the joints can go a long way toward relieving joint pain, not to mention the benefits exercise provides to overall endurance, well-being, and mood. Two exercise modalities worth checking out are tai chi, a very gentle form of martial arts that involves soft, flowing movements and no stress on the joints, and water aerobics, which can be done at different levels of difficulty without putting any stress on the joints.

For more ideas, the www.about.com website has an excellent introduction to exercise with arthritis. And if you or someone you love is truly unable to get out of a chair, there's still hope—the Sit and Be Fit program is a wonderful resource. Check it out at www.sitandbefit.org.

Natural Prescription for Arthritis

Glucosamine from glucosamine sulfate (glucosamine hydrochloride if you're allergic to sulfate or shellfish): 1,500 mg per day in divided doses (okay to take 3,000 mg a day for the first month)

Chondroitin sulfate: 1,200 to 1,500 mg (okay to reduce to 500 mg per day if you like, after the first few months)

MSM: 1,000 to 4,000 mg

Omega-3 fish oil (or essential fatty acids):
1 to 5 g (1,000 to 5,000 mg)

BSP (shea nut oil): 3 caps per day

Exercise: Water aerobics or tai chi

Note: The above dosages are daily and in pill or capsule form unless otherwise noted.

Asthma

Breathe Easier with Quercetin and Antioxidants

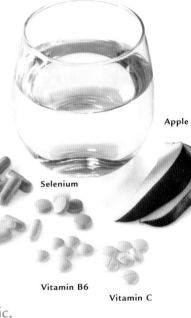

Water

Apple

Quercetin

Selenium

Magnesium

Vitamin B6

Vitamin C

CONVENTIONAL medications are often helpful for treating acute asthma attacks and for preventing recurrences. However, despite the best that modern medicine has to offer, many patients continue to experience acute attacks and/or chronic, low-level breathing difficulties. Moreover, most of the medications used to treat asthma can cause side effects. New ideas are needed if we are to win the battle against asthma.

—Jonathan Wright, M.D., co-author of
Natural Medicine, Optimal Wellness

If you've ever seen someone having an asthma attack, you know it's not pretty.

And according to those who suffer from them, an attack can be one of the scariest experiences in life. Muscles around the sufferer's airways tighten up, less air can get in, inflammation increases, the airways become even more swollen and narrow, and it becomes harder and harder to breathe. During a bad attack, the person with asthma may literally feel like he's suffocating and can't breathe. In severe cases, the airways can close so much that not enough oxygen gets to the vital organs—at which point it's a full-blown medical emergency.

You can die from that kind of attack, and approximately 4,000 to 5,000 people a year do just that. And asthma is a contributing factor to 7,000 other deaths each year.

What Is Asthma?

Asthma comes from Greek words meaning either "panting" or "sharp breath." It's a chronic disease affecting the pathways that carry air in and out of the lungs. Those airways become inflamed and sensitive to a variety of substances (in air, food, or the environment) that are irritating or allergenic. That's one reason asthma is so often linked to allergies.

Asthma is widely understood by almost everyone to be an immunological problem. The immune system mistakenly identifies substances—pollens, dust, dander, foods, etc.—as being dangerous and overreacts, setting up a cascade of events that leads to inflammation in the lungs and a narrowing of the air passages.

If that overreaction of the immune system to everyday stimuli sounds somewhat like the description of an allergy, it's because they're not entirely dissimilar. Allergic asthma is a specific type of asthma that can be triggered by an allergy to, for example, pollen or mold. And it's common: In the United States, it's estimated that about half of asthma sufferers have allergic asthma.

Because allergies (and asthma) are inflammatory disorders, it makes sense that a diet high in natural anti-inflammatory agents (e.g., vegetables and some fruits) is going to be a good idea for sufferers. And for asthma—and allergies—one of the best and most powerful of the natural anti-inflammatories is a substance called *quercetin*.

The Most Important Flavonoid

In the coloring of fruits and vegetables there are thousands of molecules known collectively as *polyphenols*. One particular class of these polyphenols is called *flavonoids*. And the most abundant, most bioavailable, and most studied of these flavonoids is a compound called *quercetin*.

Quercetin—which was called "the most important flavonoid" by the peer-reviewed journal *Nutrition in Cancer*—is anti-inflammatory, making it useful in helping to calm the symptoms of asthma (and allergies). It's found in onions, apples, berries, tea, red wine, and supplements. In one study published in 2002 in the *American Journal of Clinical Nutrition*, higher quercetin intakes were associated with a lower incidence of asthma.

"Quercetin has a very unique molecular structure," says David Nieman, Ph.D., author of *Nutritional Assessment* and head of the Appalachian State University Human Performance Lab. "It has many effects in humans. It impacts the immune system, it reacts against cancer cells, and it's a powerful anti-inflammatory."

In the voluminous literature linking dietary habits and disease, quercetin has an impressive history of being linked to a reduction in heart disease as well as to a reduction in lung cancer. Epidemiological studies have suggested that high consumption of apples may protect against asthma, and quercetin may be the main reason why.

The quercetin in the apple is, interestingly enough, in the peel. "The peel prevents the harmful effects of the UV rays of the sun from hurting the fruit," Nieman says. "It also prevents microbes from getting in. So quercetin is the first line of defense for the apple. It appears to have many of these same protective effects on human cells."

One of the reasons quercetin is so helpful with asthma (and allergies) has to do with cells in the body known as mast cells. Mast cells are responsible for a lot of the crummy symptoms you have when you get an allergy attack or experience asthmatic wheezing. The mast cells, which are actually part of the immune system, carry around all sorts of granules, the most famous of which is histamine. During an attack—of allergies or asthma—the mast cells release histamine and other chemicals like cytokines and leukotrines, causing the characteristic symptoms that drive everyone, especially the sufferer, crazy. Quercetin stabilizes the mast cells, calming them down. When you put quercetin in a test tube with mast cells, they relax. And that's exactly what you want, whether you're suffering from an allergy attack, asthmatic wheezing, or both.

WORTH KNOWING

Quercetin is widely available as a supplement. One quercetin supplement that I recommend highly is a mix of quercetin and bromelain called the A.I. Formula by Pure Encapsulations. It's available on my website, www.jonny-bowden.com.

Asthma and Allergies: Overlapping Components

Asthma and allergies share a relationship to emotional stress. Even conventional doctors, especially the younger ones, now know that asthma has significant emotional triggers in addition to its physical components. Anxiety and stress are common asthma triggers—just as they are for so many other conditions and symptoms. It's not that emotions cause asthma, but they can make symptoms a lot worse. Strong emotions can even trigger an attack.

Stress management may be one of the best natural cures, or adjuncts, for managing asthma severity. Learn to recognize both thought patterns and behavior patterns that are stressful for you and develop techniques for cutting them off at the pass.

Image therapy is a method of treating asthma that was devised by a psychologist named Elizabeth Shafer who herself suffered from debilitating asthma. Image therapy can help prevent you from panicking or stressing out at the first sign of an asthma event, which only makes everything worse. Buteyko therapy, which teaches a different way of breathing, is also worth looking into.

Food Allergies and Sensitivities

Although external environmental substances (like pollen) can trigger some asthma, food can also trigger or exacerbate the condition. According to Alan Gaby, M.D., an unrecognized food allergy (and/or food intolerance) is a contributing factor in at least 75 percent of people with childhood asthma and about 40 percent of those with adult asthma.

"As early as 1959, Albert H. Rowe, M.D., a pioneer in the field of food allergy, successfully treated 95 asthmatic patients with dietary changes alone," Gaby says. At the top of the list of foods most likely to provoke asthma? Dairy products. Other usual suspects include eggs, chocolate, wheat, corn, citrus fruits, and fish. Tartrazine (yellow dye #5) is believed to be a trigger for thousands of people.

The Stomach Acid Connection

One reason why food sensitivities and asthma show up together so often can be found in a study done decades ago by George Bray, M.D., and it has to do with stomach acid. In 1931, Bray compared children with and without asthma and found that while only one out of five non-asthmatic children was deficient in

Natural Prescription for Asthma

Quercetin: 500 mg, twice a day (preferably taken with bromelain)

Magnesium: 300 to 600 mg

Vitamin B6: 50 to 200 mg

Vitamin C: 1,000 to 3,000 mg

Selenium: 200 mcg

Note: All dosages are daily dosages and in pill or capsule form unless otherwise noted.

hydrochloric acid (HCl), four out of five of the asthmatic kids were. Low levels of HCl can significantly impair digestion and can increase allergies—or sensitivities—to foods.

In Bray's study, when the low-acid kids were given HCl before or during meals and still avoided trigger foods, they had noticeable improvements in asthmatic attacks, and the attacks became shorter and less severe.

Selenium and Vitamin C: The Powerhouse Antioxidants

People with asthma are subjected to increased oxidative stress, the damage done to cells by free radicals of oxygen molecules. One super antioxidant that has special importance to people with asthma is *selenium*. A number of studies have revealed low selenium levels in people with asthma, and one study—in the *American Journal of Respiratory and Critical Care Medicine*—reported that study participants with the highest intakes of selenium were only about half as likely to have asthma as those who consumed the least. (Not much selenium was needed for the positive effect—less than 100 mcg.) The researchers suggested that part of the blame for Britain's rising asthma rate might be the nation's declining selenium intake.

Asthmatics have a higher need for vitamin C than do members of the general population. Low intakes of vitamin C from food or supplementation can lead to increased risks for asthma. One to two grams of vitamin C have been shown in studies to be the most helpful for asthmatics. Higher intakes (and blood levels) of vitamin C are related to decreased levels of histamine production.

Other supplements that may help with asthma include magnesium and vitamin B6. Low levels of B6 and magnesium are frequently found together with asthma, and some research has shown improvement in the frequency and severity of asthma symptoms with magnesium and B6 supplementation.

Bad Breath

Clear the Air with Digestive Enzymes and Probiotics

BAD BREATH is another fine example of how the body has a limited number of ways to respond to an infinite number of "insults" or problems. The conventional wisdom is that it's caused by something in the mouth—poor oral hygiene, for example. But just as skin blemishes are only sometimes a surface issue and more commonly stem from something systemic, bad breath only sometimes comes from the mouth.

Hydrogen Peroxide

Charcoal Tablets

Probiotics

Oil of Oregano

A great deal of bad breath actually originates in the gut. Poor digestion is a frequent culprit. Enter digestive enzymes. Digestive enzymes that contain hydrochloric acid (HCl) would probably benefit most people over forty regardless of whether they have bad breath. Not only do they address some of the causes of bad breath at the root, they also help us break down and use protein, which can become a lot more difficult for people over forty. Many folks don't make sufficient HCl to adequately break down protein and other foods, so a capsule that combines digestive enzymes and HCl is highly recommended.

Many holistic physicians and health practitioners have recently written about the myriad health problems associated with low stomach acid. Bad breath, bloating, gas, and even fatigue are among the many symptoms of low stomach acid, which HCl can help.

A great way to determine how much HCl you need is this: Take one HCl capsule before a big meal. At the next big meal, take two capsules, and at the third big meal take three capsules, and so on. Continue to do this until you feel a warming sensation in your stomach. Then back off one capsule, and that is the dosage you need to help you with digestion.

Gut health depends on the proper balance of bacteria, so if you suspect digestive problems are at the root of bad breath, a good probiotic supplement—acidophilus and/or bifidus—is a great idea. Fructoogliosaccharides (FOS)—a particularly healthy form of nondigestible carbohydrates—are sometimes included in such formulations because they act as food for the "good bugs."

A Diet for Bad Breath

When gut ecology is not properly balanced between the "good" and the "bad" bacteria, it's like having a garden that's overgrown with weeds. The weeds in this case are bacteria like Candida albicans (yeast), which can cause all sorts of health problems, not the least of which is really bad breath. Oil of oregano capsules are a great way to kill the little buggers.

You also want to starve them. Since they live on sugar, an "anti-yeast" diet—something like the early stages of the Atkins Diet, with no sugar, bread, pasta, rice, cereal, or even fruit for a couple of weeks—is just the ticket. Protein, vegetables, and good fats such as olive oil are the way to go.

Activated charcoal is another great supplement that can help with odors and even toxins originating in the gut. It may also sweeten your breath. Chlorophyll is nature's deodorizer and, according to some naturopaths, a great blood purifier, meaning it helps support detoxification. The popular breath-freshening gum Clorets capitalized on this connection between chlorophyll and deodorizing, but truth be told, chlorophyll packs a powerful wallop. Some practitioners recommend taking a few capsules or tablets on an empty stomach to support gut health and detoxification. And more fiber in your diet—always a good idea—promotes the elimination of toxins from the body.

The more whole foods you can incorporate into your diet the better because highly processed foods loaded with bad fats and sugar can contribute to digestive problems (and bad breath). I've long been an advocate of daily, fresh-made vegetable and fruit juice (see *The 150 Healthiest Foods on Earth*). Vegetables and fruits also help balance the system by providing a nice alkaline balance to our highly acidic, overly processed standard American diet. Alternately, some of the "green drinks" now found in health food supermarkets are a great choice and accomplish some of the same things. These drinks frequently contain nice doses of chlorophyll-containing grasses. (My favorite, available on my website www.jonnybowden.com as well as in health food groceries everywhere is Barlean's Greens.)

Natural Breath Mints

In addition to the above recommendations, herbs and spices can sweeten your breath. Try the following.

Parsley and mint. Chewing parsley or mint leaves has been a natural remedy for thousands of years. These herbs are especially good if garlic and onions are the source of your bad breath. Parsley is very high in chlorophyll. Try chewing a few parsley sprigs dipped in vinegar for immediate relief. If you swallow the leaves after chewing them they will be digested and continue to provide fresh breath for a while. These plants seem to reduce the production of intestinal gas by promoting better digestion.

Peelu is a natural twig fortified with minerals that help clean the teeth and other inhibitors that prevent gums from bleeding. It also has cleaning agents that kill microbes and germs and a scent that makes breath naturally fresh. Peelu is an ideal brush that has been naturally endowed with more breath-freshening, mouth-cleaning compounds than any artificially made toothpaste.

Finally, herbs like coriander, ginger, cumin, and fennel are helpful. Indian restaurants usually provide a little bowl of fennel seeds for customers. Chewing on them freshens the breath in the nicest and most natural way.

Natural Prescription for Bad Breath

Digestive enzymes: 1 or 2 with every meal

Probiotics: 1 or 2, three times a day or as directed. You can also take the powdered form with water.

Charcoal tablets in between meals: Activated charcoal absorbs toxins and is a natural purifier. (Take it with plenty of water, and not at the same time as nutritional supplements or medications, as it may theoretically interfere with absorption.)

Hydrogen peroxide: Gargling and rinsing with hydrogen peroxide has been found to be terrific for many people.

Oil of oregano: 2 capsules, three times a day

Green drinks: Daily

Note: All dosages are daily dosages and in pill or capsule form unless otherwise noted.

Benign Prostatic Hyperplasia (BPH)

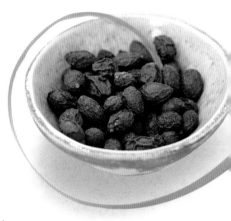

Skip the Midnight Trip to the Bathroom with Saw Palmetto

DOES WAKING UP in the middle of the night to go to the bathroom sound familiar? If you're a man over forty, chances are you've experienced the all-too-common symptoms of benign prostatic hyperplasia (BPH). Frequent urination, especially in the middle of the night, is the signature of this annoying but essentially harmless condition. So are a hesitant, interrupted, or weak stream of urine, a pressing urgency to urinate, leaking, and dribbling.

Annoying as it is, BPH is not usually dangerous. However, you need to be aware of two things. One, urine retention and strain on the bladder can lead to more serious problems, including bladder damage, kidney damage, bladder stones, urinary tract infection, and the inability to control urination. If you catch BPH early, there's a much lower risk of such complications. And fortunately, there are some easy and natural ways to bring relief (more on that in a moment).

Saw palmetto is the go-to herb when it comes to taming the urge to urinate every few hours. A three-year study in Germany found that 160 mg of saw palmetto extract taken twice daily reduced nighttime urination in 73 percent of people and improved urinary flow rates significantly. Another multi-center study showed that a similar amount treated BPH as well as the drug Proscar, but without the side effects.

Though we don't know the exact cause of BPH, it's widely believed that it's fueled by hormones, specifically testosterone and even more specifically the metabolism of testosterone. But what's even more important is what happens to the testosterone that we do make. Some testosterone is converted in the body to a nasty little metabolite called DHT (dihydrotestosterone). DHT is thought to be partly responsible for male baldness, and a high conversion of testosterone to DHT in women is thought to be connected to a host of "male" symptoms, like hair loss (on the head) and hair growth (on the face). This conversion—in both men and women—is fueled by an enzyme called 5-alpha-reductase. Saw palmetto helps to down-regulate this enzyme, meaning a reduction in the amount of DHT. Saw palmetto also contains compounds that act as anti-inflammatories.

Note: It's always good to rule out cancer as a cause of the urinary symptoms. A blood test called a PSA (for prostate-specific antigen) is a good idea. Though the test is hardly conclusive for cancer, PSA is frequently elevated in the blood of men with prostate cancer.

Other Helpful Supplements

Although saw palmetto is the superstar nutrient for "curing" all-night bathroom breaks, four other supplements have also been found to be helpful.

Pygeum is an extract from the bark of an African tree and is approved in at least three countries in Europe as a BPH remedy. It relieves symptoms of BPH and contains at least three types of compounds (including beta-sitosterol, listed below) that help the prostate.

Beta-sitosterol is a plant sterol found in almost all plants, especially in rice bran, wheat germ, corn oils, and soybeans. In clinical research it's been shown to help lower blood cholesterol, but more to the point, it's also been shown to reduce the symptoms of BPH. Four double-blind, placebo-controlled studies including 519 men and lasting from 4 to 26 weeks concluded that beta-sitosterol significantly improved urological symptoms and flow measures.

Nettles (stinging nettles) are frequently combined with other "prostate herbs" like saw palmetto and have long been believed to have a beneficial effect on prostate health. One recent double-blind, placebo-controlled study in a 2005 issue of the *Journal of Herb Pharmacotherapy* found that it had beneficial effects, and other studies have also been encouraging.

Pumpkin seeds have a well-deserved reputation as a prostate-friendly food and are an approved "therapy" for men with BPH in Germany. In a few studies, pumpkin-seed oil has been shown to have a good effect on BPH symptoms, but no good research shows that they work by themselves. You can use pumpkin extract in combination with saw palmetto in supplements for prostate health.

Although the research on zinc for BPH is spotty, most complementary and holistic health practitioners recommend it. Zinc is absolutely essential to prostate health. Prostatic secretions contain a high concentration of zinc. Zinc also tones down the activity of the 5-alpha-reductase enzyme, which, you may recall, fuels the conversion of testosterone to dihydrotestosterone. (And let's not forget that stress depletes zinc like crazy, so many individuals may have low levels to begin with.)

"Whatever you do, if you have an enlarged prostate along with the usual symptoms, don't reach for that saw palmetto without picking up the zinc and essential fatty acids, too," says the noted teacher of nutritional medicine Alan Gaby, M.D. Gaby and others usually recommend beginning with a large amount of zinc (typically 50 to 100 mg a day). Since that dose of zinc can conceivably lead to an imbalance in copper, Gaby and others also add 2 to 4 mg of copper. "After several months, the dose is typically reduced to 30 mg once or twice a day, depending on the patient's response," says Gaby. The best-absorbed forms of zinc are zinc picolinate and zinc citrate.

Natural Prescription for Benign Prostate Hyperplasia

Saw palmetto: 320 mg (160 mg, twice a day)

CAN BE COMBINED WITH (APPROXIMATE VALUES):

Pygeum: 100 to 200 mg (50 to 100 mg, twice a day)

Stinging nettles: 300 mg (150 mg, twice a day)

Beta-sitosterol: 100 to 300 mg (150 mg, twice a day)

Zinc: 50 mg to start; reduce to 30 mg after a few months

Note: All dosages are daily dosages and in pill or capsule form unless otherwise noted.

Cravings

Calm Your Appetite for Carbs with Glutamine

NEXT TIME a carbohydrate urge hits, reach for the white stuff. No, not granulated sugar. *Glutamine*. L-glutamine (also known as glutamine) is the most abundant amino acid in the human body. We store the majority of it in our muscles and use it up in heavy exercise, which is why it's such a popular supplement among bodybuilders and athletes. (It's also critical for the immune system; one of the reasons marathoners frequently get sick after the event is that so much glutamine is used up during intense exercise.) Glutamine's also a very important nutrient for intestinal health and wound healing. And glutamine can help with cravings. For both sugar *and* alcohol.

The Atkins Connection

I first learned about using glutamine from Robert Atkins, M.D., who actually learned about it from Roger Williams, M.D. Williams, a pioneer in nutritional medicine, was the father of the term *biochemical individuality* and the author of several books on nutrition and alcohol. He was one of the first to recognize the deep and intimate connection between cravings for alcohol and cravings for sugar, and he used glutamine for both.

It started back in the 1950s, when Williams did an experiment with alcohol-loving rats. First he established which rats liked to drink by giving them the opportunity to drink freely from either of two bottles—one filled with tap water and one containing 10 percent alcohol. Then he picked nineteen rats that tended to like the alcohol the most, and divided them into two groups. One group received 100 mg of L-glutamine mixed with their food, the other group didn't.

At the end of 17 days, he returned all the rats to a regular diet of Purina rat chow and watched and measured what they drank.

The rats fed the glutamine consumed, on the whole, 35 percent less alcohol over the next nine days than the rats that were not fed the glutamine. Williams concluded that "glutamine administered orally appears to be a relatively effective agent in decreasing the voluntary consumption of alcohol by rats."

It also seems to work on humans. In a study published in the *Quarterly Journal of Studies on Alcohol* in 1957, Williams found that 1 g of L-glutamine in divided doses with meals significantly reduced both cravings and the anxiety that accompanies alcohol withdrawal. In another experiment, a daily dose of about 3 teaspoons did the trick for about three-quarters of the people studied. Why these studies were never followed up on amazes me, but glutamine continues to be used by many knowledgeable practitioners who work with both alcoholics and sugar addicts, and it's used in many alcoholism programs across the country.

Cure Those Constant Cravings

When you experience a craving, it's because your brain wants sugar. And it wants it now! Glutamine is an alternate source of glucose available to the brain, plus it has the added advantage of getting there quickly! You can open a capsule and put it under your tongue and you'll feel the crave-reducing effect within minutes. Or better yet, put a heaping spoonful in water.

"[Glutamine] provides a ready source of brain fuel for hypoglycemics and helps stave off sugar cravings … that develop when blood sugar levels drop too low," says Joan Mathews-Larson, Ph.D, director of the excellent program for addicts at the Health Recovery Center in Minneapolis.

Abram Hoffer, M.D., Ph.D., a Canadian psychiatrist and one of the pioneers in the practice of orthomolecular medicine (the practice of using megavitamins and nutrients to treat disease) called L-glutamine "an amino acid that decreases physiological cravings for alcohol" and "one of the two primary energy providers that … provide fuel to the brain."

Atkins has suggested the following for a sugar urge: Take 1 to 2 g of L-glutamine, preferably with some heavy cream and just a touch of nonsugar

Natural Prescription for Cravings

Take 1 heaping teaspoon of glutamine powder dissolved in water when a craving strikes or as a preventive measure (preferably on an empty stomach). Alternately, take three or four times a day, in between meals.

Note: The above dosages are daily dosages and in pill or capsule form, unless otherwise noted.

sweetener. "The immediate desire to eat something sweet will pass," he said. "For a reference attesting to its efficiency, ask any of the 8,000 Atkins Center patients for whom I have prescribed it!"

Depression
Feel Better with These Natural Antidepressants

CONSIDER THIS: You're lying on the couch, unable to motivate yourself enough to get up and get dressed. Everything seems pointless, hopeless, and dark, and all you want to do is stare into space. There's a pill sitting on the coffee table a few feet in front of you that promises to make you feel 100 percent better and take your depression away. And you can't muster the enthusiasm or energy to get up and get it.

That's the best—and truest—description of severe depression I've ever heard. I remember recognizing it instantly as being a perfect description of the hell that is depression.

I know, because it's exactly how I felt for one horrendous year in my life, right after I moved to Los Angeles and promptly got divorced.

Luckily, it didn't last (feeling horrendous, that is—the divorce has gone quite well, thank you). And yes, I did use a pharmaceutical prescription—Lexapro, actually—to help get up off the couch and put some things into motion that actually helped me get rid of the depression. But I haven't used Lexapro for years, and I've seen plenty of other people get off antidepressants—or avoid going on them in the first place—by using a combination of natural substances from amino acids to St. John's Wort. One of the best of those natural substances is 5-HTP.

Depression Is Not a Prozac Deficiency

The term 5-HTP stands for 5-hydroxytryptophan, and it's the stuff out of which your body makes serotonin, one of the major players in a group of neurotransmitters—chemicals that transmit information in the brain. Though depression is complicated and undoubtedly has many precipitating factors, it's widely accepted that neurotransmitters are deeply involved, especially serotonin. Low levels of serotonin are associated with cravings, anxiety, obsessive-compulsive disorder, aggressive behavior, and depression.

We don't know exactly how all the neurotransmitters work together to cause or affect depression in all its many forms, but we do suspect that low levels of serotonin play a big part in what people experience as depression.

It's not for nothing that serotonin is known as the "feel good" neurotransmitter. Without enough of it we don't do very well. The most popular pharmaceutical antidepressants—Prozac, Zoloft, Lexapro, etc.—belong to a class called serotonin selective reuptake inhibitors (SSRIs). The SSRIs do just what the term says—they inhibit the action of the cleanup crew that "mops up" serotonin from the brain, thus allowing serotonin to hang around longer. The more serotonin, goes the reasoning, the happier the camper.

Enter 5-HTP. Your body makes serotonin from an amino acid known as L-tryptophan. L-tryptophan is an amino acid, found in protein foods like meat and seafood. The body turns tryptophan it into a metabolite called 5-HTP (5-hydroxytryptophan) and then, with the help of vitamin B6, into 5-HT (5-hydroxytryptamine), better known to all of us as plain old serotonin.

One Step Away from Serotonin

For years health practitioners had used tryptophan to help people sleep and as a natural aid to relaxation and calm. A lot of people were very upset when it was taken off the market. But lucky for us, 5-HTP is even better. As explained above, it's only one step from 5-HTP to serotonin. In addition, in animal and human studies, 5-HTP, unlike tryptophan, has been demonstrated to increase catecholamine metabolism, specifically working on dopamine and norepinephrine— other "feel-good" neurotransmitters that are involved in mood. (It's possible that the antidepressant effect of 5-HTP may be related to a combined effect on serotonin and other neurotransmitters.) Regardless of its effect on other brain chemicals, supplemental 5-HTP surely increases serotonin, and because of that, has a calming, relaxing effect on brain chemistry. It's used for mild and moderate depression and it also may help you sleep better. Why? Because at night, serotonin converts into melatonin, which is important for a great night's sleep.

For some people, 5-HTP may perform equally to or better than standard antidepressant drugs and in most cases, without side effects. One study compared 5-HTP to fluvoxamine (brand name Luvox), an SSRI like Prozac,

Paxil, and Zoloft. In the study, subjects received either 5-HTP (100 mg) or fluvoxamine (50 mg) three times daily for six weeks. More patients felt better after using 5-HTP than fluvoxamine, and 5-HTP was quicker acting than the fluvoxamine. And in one other study, patients who were unresponsive to other antidepressant therapy showed significant improvement when using 5-HTP.

Listen, I'm the last person to tell you to throw out your pharmaceutical antidepressants. I believe they've helped many people—including me—and probably saved a lot of lives. But if you have mild or moderate depression, or any of the other conditions mentioned above that might respond to a boost in the brain chemical serotonin, you might give 5-HTP a try. And if you're lucky—and many people are—you may find that by using 5-HTP, you may not need the "big guns" at all.

St. Johns Wort: An Historic and Helpful Herb

St. John's Wort is actually a perennial herb with many flowers that can be found growing wild in much of the world (the word "wort" just means plant). It's got a long and honorable history of use, probably dating back to the ancient Greeks, who believed that the fragrance of St. John's Wort caused evil spirits to simply fly, fly away. (Okay, maybe these days, not so much.)

But it does have a 2,400-year history of folk use for everything from anxiety to sleep disturbances. St. John's Wort was officially recognized as an antidepressant drug in Germany in 1998, is covered by the country's national health-care system, and in fact is the number one prescribed antidepressant in Germany and most of Europe.

Supported by Studies

A meta-analysis published in the *British Medical Journal* in 1996 reviewed 23 published trials on St. John's Wort involving more than 1,700 patients. The researchers, lead by Klaus Linde, M.D., reported findings that extracts of St. John's Wort were more effective than a placebo for the treatment of mild to moderately severe depression. The authors emphasized that it's not yet known whether the extracts are more effective for some types of depression than others, but that certainly looks to be the case.

It's worth noting that overall, only about 10 percent of the patients in the studies had side effects with St. John's Wort (like dry mouth, allergic reactions, and some gastrointestinal upset), compared with about 35 percent

WORTH KNOWING

There's a lack of info about the effects of taking 5-HTP during pregnancy, so check with your health professional or be on the safe side and don't use it. It can affect prolactin, a hormone necessary for milk production, so it might be a good idea to avoid it while breastfeeding. Because it does increase serotonin, it's wise to check with a knowledgeable health care professional about possible interactions with other drugs or supplements. Really. Though 5-HTP is great stuff, don't start mixing and matching with pharmaceuticals or taking yourself off medications without your doctor's knowledge. It can be done, but do it wisely and with supervision.

of patients who reported side effects from prescription antidepressants. Only about 5 percent of the patients stopped taking it because of side effects, a low number indeed.

Many other studies have shown St. John's Wort to be effective, and with virtually no significant side effects (more on that in a moment). Another 1999 study, also published in the *British Medical Journal*, tested hypericin extract—one of the active ingredients in St. John's Wort—against both a placebo and a standard antidepressant (imipramine) in a randomized, multi-center study involving 263 patients with moderate depression. Hypericin was more effective than the placebo at reducing depression (as measured by

WORTH KNOWING

The best preparation seems to be the St. John's Wort extract standardized to contain 0.3 percent hypericin, and the recommended dosage of this as an antidepressant is 300 mg, taken three times a day, close to meals. You can also drink it as a tea (boiling water poured onto one to two teaspoons of the dried herb, infused for 10 to 15 minutes).

St. John's Wort interacts with a lot of medications, so if you're on meds, check with a health professional knowledgeable about both St. John's Wort and pharmaceuticals before beginning to take it. It can also make you more sensitive to the sun, so if you like to spend time at the beach, be careful if you're on St. John's Wort.

the Hamilton depression scores and, even more dramatically, by the Zung self-rating depression scale), and performed just as well as the drug, with notably fewer side effects. The researchers noted that while both the drug and St. John's Wort improved the mental component scale of Short Form-36 (a widely used standardized test), only St. John's Wort improved the physical component scale.

"The rate of adverse events with the hypericin extract was in the range of the placebo group but lower than that of the (drug) group," researchers noted.

According to noted expert Steven Bratman, M.D., author of the excellent reference book *The Natural Pharmacy*, St. John's Wort has a scientific record approaching that of many prescription drugs, and is effective in about 55 percent of cases. Bratman also points out that there is good evidence that it's at least as effective as fluoxetine (Prozac) and sertraline (Zoloft). If you're feeling mild symptoms of depression, St. John's Wort is definitely worth a try.

SAMe: A Natural Cure for Depression

SAMe is arguably the most effective "natural" antidepressant around. And one of the best things about it is that you'll know whether it's working within a week, (although in some much less common cases it may take up to five weeks to work, about the same as a pharmaceutical antidepressant in the SSRI class.)

SAMe is not a vitamin nor an herb, but a naturally occurring molecule that all living cells (including ours) produce.

In treating depression, SAMe works as well as certain standard antidepressants* and with fewer side effects. In a meta-analysis of twenty-eight studies done by the Agency for Healthcare Research and Quality, treatment

Natural Prescription for Depression

5-HTP: Start with 50 mg three times a day and increase if necessary after two weeks. A common dose for depression and headache is
300 mg daily.

OR

St. John's Wort: 300 mg, standardized for 0.3 percent

Hypericin: Three times a day

Note: All dosages are daily dosages and in pill or capsule form unless otherwise noted.

OR

SAMe: 800 mg a day in two doses (400 mg in the a.m., 400 mg in the p.m.)

Note: Do not take SAMe if you're suffering from bipolar disorder

In addition:

Omega-3 fatty acids: 1 to 3 g daily

Remove sugar from diet

Exercise daily!

FOR ADDED EFFECTIVENESS:

Inositol: 612 g for as long as needed

Note: The above dosages are daily and in pill or capsule form unless otherwise noted.

with SAMe was associated with an improvement of about six points on the Hamilton Rating Scale for Depression after only three weeks, basically equal to treatment with conventional antidepressants and significantly better than treatment with a placebo. A paper in *Psychiatry Research* (1995) from researchers at the Depression Clinical and Research Program at Massachusetts General Hospital concluded that "SAMe is a relatively safe and fast-acting antidepressant." A review of the evidence published in the *American Journal of Clinical Nutrition* in 2002 by two researchers affiliated with Harvard Medical School (Mischoulon and Fava) pointed out that SAMe may have a faster onset of action than conventional antidepressants and may even protect against the deleterious effects of Alzheimer's. This is good stuff.

A review of eleven research papers on SAMe, published in *Clinical Investigative Medicine* in June 2005, concluded that "there appears to be a role for SAMe in the treatment of major depression in adults." Note the qualifier "major." It's extremely hard to treat "major" depression, so the fact that the researchers were positive about SAMe says more than you might think on first glance. "Major depression" is one of three categories of depression, but if you're reading this—and you're depressed—chances are you don't have "major" depression but instead have either "mild" or "moderate" depression, both of which respond even better to SAMe. About 70 percent of people with depression respond to SAMe, according to Richard Brown, M.D., author of *Stop Depression Now*.

Depression accompanies a lot of health conditions. People with diabetes, fibromyalgia, Parkinson's disease, and other illnesses frequently suffer from depression, often at a higher rate than the general population. SAMe is a valuable tool for treating depression in these folks, especially because there are no reported adverse interactions with SAMe and other drugs, dietary supplements, or foods.

Though 5-HTP, St. Johns Wort, and SAMe are all wonderful, don't try all three at once. Give each one a real shot of a few weeks and then, if it's not working, try one of the others.

Diabetes/Metabolic Syndrome

Start with Chromium and Skip the Carbs

TYPE 2 DIABETES is a chronic condition in which the body's ability to metabolize sugar is impaired. Though it was once known as "adult-onset diabetes," it has been showing up in younger and younger people over the past two decades. Each year, according to the Centers for Disease Control and Prevention (CDC), more than 13,000 young people are diagnosed with it, a number likely to grow even larger over the next few decades.

It's impossible to talk about diabetes—and its relative, metabolic syndrome (also known as pre-diabetes)—without discussing a hormone called insulin.

In a nutshell, here's what happens: When you eat, your blood sugar goes up. In response to this elevated blood sugar, the pancreas makes a hormone called insulin, whose many jobs in the body include whisking that extra sugar out of the bloodstream and into the cells where it can be burned for energy.

In at least one in four people (much more by some estimates), this mechanism doesn't work properly. The cells stop paying attention to insulin, becoming resistant to its effects. This condition, called "insulin resistance," is a prominent feature of type 2 diabetes as well as metabolic syndrome—a collection of symptoms like abdominal obesity and high blood pressure that together significantly increase the risk for heart disease. The vast majority of individuals with cardiovascular disease and/or type 2 diabetes are also insulin resistant.

Start with a Low-Carb Diet

Because diabetics and people who are insulin resistant have trouble clearing sugar from their bloodstream, it makes sense that a low-sugar (also known as low-glycemic) diet would be helpful as it would lessen the load on an already dysfunctional system. This is precisely the thinking that led many researchers to investigate the effects of low-carbohydrate diets on both insulin resistance and "glucose control," which is the ability of the body to keep blood sugar levels in a reasonable range. The overwhelming majority of such studies show great improvement in insulin levels and blood sugar control. My friend Barry Sears, Ph.D., often says that insulin resistance can be reversed within three days with proper diet, and the research has backed him up.

I am a huge proponent of low-carb diets, especially for anyone with insulin resistance, diabetes or metabolic syndrome (see my book, *Living Low Carb: Controlled Carbohydrate Eating for Long-Term Weight Loss*). A low-carb diet should be the first thing you try if you've got abdominal obesity, insulin resistance, or even full-blown diabetes. Many risk factors for heart disease, like high triglycerides, come plummeting down with a low-carb diet, and you will be much more able to keep blood sugar and insulin levels in control.

Chromium: Insulin's Little Helper

Chromium is a trace mineral that is directly involved in carbohydrate, fat, and protein metabolism. It's also known to enhance the action of insulin, helping it to do its job better (and therefore reducing the amount needed to get the job done).

In this way, insulin works much like certain "insulin-sensitizing" medications, such as glucophage. It literally helps open the doors of the cells so that insulin (and sugar) can get in, thus reducing the burden on the body of having high amounts of both blood sugar and insulin. According to Georgetown University Medical Center professor Harry Preuss, M.D., C.N.S., chromium activates the enzyme tyrosine kinase, which helps insulin attach to insulin receptors. It's like a key to the cell door.

The leading chromium researcher in the world is Richard Anderson, Ph.D., at the U.S. Department of Agriculture. Anderson has done a number of studies on diabetics that show their blood sugar levels dropping with chromium supplementation, particularly at the higher doses (800 to 1,000 mcg per day). Chromium has also been shown to be helpful in the treatment of gestational diabetes and may even be of some help in type 1 diabetes. In one study, even 200 mcg of chromium given to people with type 1 diabetes allowed them to reduce their average insulin dosage by almost one-third.

Simply put, chromium is "insulin's little helper."

Just one year after a typically behind-the-curve statement by the American Diabetes Association, which stated that "chromium supplementation has no known benefit in patients who are not chromium deficient," a study published in the journal *Diabetes* reached the opposite conclusion.

Researchers divided 180 people with type 2 diabetes into three groups—one group received 200 mcg of chromium picolinate a day, one group received 1,000 mcg, and the third group got a placebo. Supplemental chromium was shown to have dramatic effects on glucose and insulin variables and "significant, sustained reductions in diabetic symptoms were especially noted in those who received 1,000 mcg per day."

Dosing the Deficiency

Remember that we don't absorb chromium very well and we don't get a lot of it in our diet (the main source is brewer's yeast, liver, and of course, beer—not the way you'd want to get it if you struggle with blood sugar and weight issues). Some studies have shown no effect of chromium on blood sugar or other diabetic measures, but Anderson and other experts have pointed out that this is probably because researchers have not always used the most effective forms of chromium, or the right dosages. Anderson himself is partial to chromium picolinate, while other experts, like Preuss, favor niacin-bound chromium (chromium polynicotinate or chromium nicotinate, sold under the brand name ChromeMate). There's also GTF chromium (GTF stands for *glucose tolerance factor*), but this is a mislabeling and a misconception; no such substance exists.

Interestingly, a diet high in sugar and processed foods actually drains chromium from the body, so the paradox is that those who need it the most have the least of it. Infection, pregnancy, and stress may also reduce levels. Even those eating a lot of healthy foods like seeds, nuts, and grains may be low in chromium because many of these foods, especially soy, contain phytic acid, which decreases the absorption of chromium (and other minerals).

The main thing we can hang our hat on is chromium's ability to help lower blood sugar and make insulin work more effectively. That alone makes it a hugely important addition to the regime of anyone trying to regulate his or her blood sugar and reduce insulin resistance.

Don't confuse chromium the supplement with the dangerous form of metal that was poisoning the town in the movie Erin Brockovich. That was *hexavalent* chromium, and it is indeed a poison. *Trivalent* chromium, the kind in food and supplements, is amazingly safe. So few adverse effects have been reported that the Institute of Medicine has never established a tolerable upper intake level for it. According to Preuss, rats fed trivalent chromium at levels thousands of times higher than the reference dose for humans, based on body weight, didn't show any toxic effects.

Magnificent Magnesium

Magnesium plays a crucial role in carbohydrate metabolism. It also plays a critical role in the secretion and action of insulin, thereby helping to control blood sugar. Magnesium supplements are absolutely essential for anyone with type 2 diabetes or anyone at risk for it.

In two of the most respected, long-range studies of health ever done, the Nurses' Health Study and the Health Professionals Follow-Up Study, more than 125,000 participants with no history of diabetes, cardiovascular disease, or cancer were investigated specifically for the purpose of examining risk factors for type 2 diabetes. Over time, the risk for developing type 2 diabetes was significantly greater in both men and women with a lower intake of magnesium.

This relationship between low magnesium and diabetes has been confirmed in other research as well. In the Women's Health Study, researchers looked at the association between magnesium intake and the incidence of type 2 diabetes over an average of six years. Among overweight women, the risk of developing the disease was significantly greater among those with lower intakes of magnesium.

The Iowa Women's Study followed 40,000 women for more than six years and also examined the relationship between diabetes and magnesium. The findings suggest that a greater intake of whole grains, dietary fiber, and yes, magnesium, decreased the risk of developing type 2 diabetes in older women.

And a number of studies have looked at the potential benefits of magnesium supplements for helping to control type 2 diabetes. In one study, sixty-three subjects with below normal blood levels of magnesium received either 300 mg of elemental magnesium a day or a placebo. At the end of only sixteen weeks, those who received the magnesium had improved metabolic control of diabetes (i.e., lower levels of hemoglobin A1c, an important marker for diabetes).

Alpha Lipoic Acid: The Superstar Antioxidant

Alpha lipoic acid (ALA) is a naturally occurring compound that is made in tiny amounts in the human body. It's one of the most potent antioxidants on the planet, with two special properties that make it unique. One, it is both fat soluble and water soluble, which makes it more effective against a wide range of free radicals than say vitamin C (water-soluble only) or vitamin E (fat-soluble only). Two, it helps "recycle" those potent antioxidants (vitamins C and E).

Its activity as a super-antioxidant is part of what makes it of great interest to type 2 diabetics. Research has shown that oxidative stress (damage from free radicals) can significantly contribute to insulin resistance. ALA, in addition to its power as an antioxidant, also helps lower blood sugar and improve insulin sensitivity.

In at least four studies, ALA used orally or intravenously improved insulin sensitivity and glucose disposal in patients with type 2 diabetes. Patients who took 600 to 1,800 mg orally or 500 to 1,000 mg intravenously of ALA daily had significant improvement in insulin resistance and glucose effectiveness after four weeks of oral treatment (or after one to ten days of intravenous administration). It's also good for peripheral neuropathy, a common complication of diabetes that causes painful sensations, especially in the feet and legs. Giving ALA orally or intravenously in 600 to 1,200 mg doses each day seems to reduce symptoms such as burning, pain, numbness, and prickling of the feet and legs.

Controversy exists over which type of ALA supplements are most effective. ALA comes in two forms, the "S" form and the "R" form; the "S" form is the chemical mirror image of the "R" form. Preliminary evidence indicates that the R form is much better absorbed. R-ALA supplements are said to be as effective as or more effective than the traditional ALA supplement (which is a mix of the two forms), based on data from animal studies.

Good Scientific Evidence

Several other natural supplements that may have positive effects on diabetes have received an "A" for "good scientific evidence" by the rigorous Natural Standard, the Authority on Integrative Medicine, an international research collaboration that systematically reviews scientific evidence on complementary and alternative medicine. These include:

- **Beta-Glucan:** Beta-glucan is a soluble fiber that has gotten a lot of attention recently for its ability to lower cholesterol. But there are now several human trials that support the use of beta-glucan for controlling blood sugar. In general, fiber slows the entrance of sugar into the blood stream, so high-fiber diets are always a good idea for people with diabetes (as well as for everyone else).

- **Ginseng:** American ginseng (panax quinquefolium) has been found in studies to lower both fasting blood sugar and post-prandial (after-eating) blood sugar.

- **Gymnema:** Gymnema sylvestre is an herb that grows in the tropical forests of India, and has long been used as a natural treatment for diabetes. There is good scientific evidence that gymnema can be useful in helping control blood sugar levels especially when used in conjunction with other oral medications.

Natural Prescription for Diabetes

Chromium: 1,000 mcg*

Cinnamon: 1/2 tsp

Magnesium: 400 to 800 mg

Biotin: 8 to 16 mg

Vitamin C: 1 to 2 g

Omega-3 fatty acids: 2 to 3 g (balance with 250 to 500 mg omega-6 fatty acids, like GLA from evening primrose oil, or take a basic essential fatty acid supplement like Omega Synergy

Alpha lipoic acid: 250 to 1,000 mg

Zinc: 25 mg

Low-carbohydrate and/or high-fiber diet

Exercise: Five days a week

*You can take a higher dosage. At the famed Tacoma Clinic in Washington, noted integrative medicine guru Jonathan Wright, M.D., frequently uses 3,000 to 4,000 mcg with his diabetic or blood sugar–challenged patients with great results.

Note: All dosages are daily dosages and in pill or capsule form unless otherwise noted.

Last But Not Least

If you are diabetic or have metabolic syndrome, you might consider looking into these other supplements:

- **Biotin:** A member of the B-vitamin family, biotin has been found to decrease insulin resistance and improve glucose tolerance. Biotin enhances insulin sensitivity and increases the activity of an enzyme called gluckinase, which is responsible for helping the liver use sugar. One study that used 9 milligrams a day of biotin reduced significant decreases in fasting blood-sugar levels in type 2 diabetics, and another did the same by using 8 to 6 grams a day. Most B-vitamin formulas include less than a milligram of biotin, but for its blood sugar lowering effect you need a lot more than that. (I have high-dose biotin on my website, www.jonnybowden.com.)

- **Fish Oil:** Though there are currently no studies showing that omega-3s (fish oil) have any significant long-term effects on glucose control or insulin resistance, fish oil can lower both blood pressure (modestly) and triglycerides, an independent risk factor for heart disease. And because diabetes, like all major degenerative diseases, has a huge inflammatory component, the fact that omega-3 fats are so highly anti-inflammatory makes them an important part of any good supplement program for diabetes.

- **Cinnamon:** Several studies support the use of cinnamon in treating diabetes. The active ingredient in cinnamon—methylhydroxychalcone polymer, or MHCP—seems to mimic insulin function, increasing the uptake of sugar by the cells and signaling certain kinds of cells to turn glucose (plain blood sugar) into glycogen (the storage form of sugar). In 2003, the Beltsville Human Nutrition Research Center worked with researchers in

Pakistan to test the effects of cinnamon on blood glucose (as well as triglycerides and cholesterol) in type 2 diabetics. They found that even one gram a day of cinnamon reduced blood sugar by 18 to 29 percent and reduced triglycerides by 23 to 30 percent.

Eczema

Clear It up with This Combo Cure

Yogurt

Probiotics

TECHNICALLY, eczema is not exactly a disease, but rather the general name given for a host of skin irritations and symptoms ranging from mild to very annoying.

Evening Primrose Oil

The two main types are contact dermatitis, which is aggravated when the skin comes in direct contact with an allergen such as household detergents and chemicals, or even cosmetics; and atopic dermatitis, which is aggravated by ingested or inhaled allergens such as certain foods, pollen, dust, or animal dander.

These external triggers ultimately irritate and strip away the outermost layer of skin—called the stratum corneum—causing moisture to escape. From there, it's a vicious cycle: The moisture escapes, which lets in more allergens, which triggers another drying reaction, and so on. The result is what we commonly call eczema. It affects 15 million Americans and nearly 10 percent of all infants and children.

Atopic dermatitis, the kind of eczema we're talking about here, is one of the first signs of allergy during infancy and is believed to be caused by delayed development of the immune system. It affects between 10 and 20 percent of all infants, but almost half of these kids will "grow out" of eczema between the ages of five and fifteen, according to the American Academy of Dermatologists.

But many won't.

Two wonderful supplements—evening primrose oil and probiotics—may help. As will one very important dietary modification (more on that in a moment).

Scratching Beneath the Surface for Causes

First understand this: Eczema can be difficult to treat partly because you have to do some detective work to figure out just which stressors may be triggering the dry, scaly skin in the first place. Meanwhile, you're fighting the overwhelming urge to scratch and rub the dry, irritated skin, which only makes it more prone to soreness and infection. The arsenal of conventional medical treatments pretty much consists of symptom-treating steroids, antihistamines, and even antibiotics. These treatments will most definitely provide short-term relief, but they in no way address the root cause of the eczema. Moreover, and especially in the case of antibiotics, they will probably do more damage to your health in the long term.

If you want to heal eczema naturally, a great place to start is by examining possible food triggers. There's a connection between atopic dermatitis and food sensitivities or allergies, and believe it or not, your food triggers can be programmed as early as in the womb. A recent study in the *American Journal of Clinical Nutrition* showed that eating certain foods during the last four weeks of pregnancy increases the risk of eczema for the infant. High intakes of vegetable oil and margarine, for example, were associated with an almost 50 percent increase in risk, while eating foods high in omega-3 fatty acids was associated with a decreased risk. (Celery—believe it or not—was associated with an 85 percent increase in risk.) And it doesn't end in the womb.

A 1990 study in the journal *Pediatrics* found that there were clear and consistent associations between eczema and the diversity of a child's diet during the first four months of life. The more variety of solid foods that a mother introduced to her baby before the age of four months old, the greater were the odds of the baby developing atopic eczema. Kids who were exposed to four or more different types of solid foods before the age of four months had almost three times the risk of recurrent or chronic eczema than those who weren't exposed to solid feeding (one more strong argument for breast milk, but that's another story).

Regardless of what your mother ate during pregnancy, remember this: Eczema is treatable, even more successfully if you take a little time to find out what triggers it. Once you identify those triggers in your diet or your child's, you can begin to eliminate or reduce them. Add in the combo cures we're about to discuss, and you're on the way to relief.

Eliminating the Triggers

Many studies have linked food allergies to eczema, so a good place to start in your detective work is with an elimination diet. (If, after using this approach, you are still stumped, it's time to move on to food allergy-food sensitivity testing, but you may not have to.)

An elimination diet is a nice, easy, low-tech way to help yourself identify which foods can be causing you problems. All you do is select a "potential offender" and then eliminate it completely from your diet for a minimum of four or five days—three weeks is even better. Then notice whether you feel better or your symptoms improve.

Obviously, this can be a long process if you go through every single food on the planet, but the fact is that most people eat about thirteen foods all the time. It might seem counterintuitive, but start with the foods you consume most frequently, even those you're "sure" couldn't be a problem because you eat them all the time.

The most common foods that exacerbate eczema are cow's milk, eggs, wheat, soy, peanuts, fish, cheese, chocolate, coloring agents, and tomatoes. When these foods are removed, eczema has been shown to go into remission. Keep in mind that we are all biochemically unique—everyone reacts differently to foods, and even though the usual suspects such as wheat, dairy, and the like may be triggers for a large number of people, there are always people who will be allergic to weirdly improbable, and sometimes extremely healthy, foods like asparagus.

With any luck you'll be one of the fortunate ones who solve the food allergy connection on the first try using an elimination diet. If you're still stumped, it may be worth the money to invest in a test that identifies food and environmental irritants to effectively solve the eczema dilemma. A good, qualified health-care practitioner can help you with the right test. Two tests worth looking into are the ALCAT test and the LEAP test. The ALCAT test is provided by Cell Science Systems Corporation in Florida and is available in more than eighteen countries as of this writing. The LEAP test (Lifestyle, Eating, and Performance) is administered by Signet Diagnostic Corporation in Florida and has an outstanding medical advisory board. To find out more about the ALCAT test, call (800) 872-5228 or go to www.alcat.com. For more information on the LEAP test, call (888) 669-5327 or go to www.nowleap.com.

If you want the simplified version of what to do—the eczema version of those "quick start" instruction sheets that come with your electronic devices—simply do this: eliminate grains (especially wheat), dairy, and sugar. Do this for a few weeks and see what happens. A surprising number of symptoms and conditions, possibly including eczema, will improve immediately by eliminating these three dietary components.

Adding in the Combos: Fats and Bugs

A common school of thought holds that eczema may be caused by the lack of—or blocking of—an important enzyme called *delta-6-desaturase*. Here's how it works: Fatty acids go through a number of metabolic transformations in the body and are the building blocks for both other fatty acids and compounds known as prostaglandins (or eicosanoids), which can be inflammatory or anti-inflammatory. (That's one reason you want the right balance of fatty acids in your diet.)

Delta-6-desaturase is one of the important enzymes that works on this fatty acid assembly line. Your body needs this enzyme to create a very important omega-6 fatty acid called *gamma-linolenic acid* (GLA). Too little delta-6-desaturase, too little GLA. And GLA has been shown to be highly beneficial in the treatment of eczema, leading many to believe that not having enough of it could aggravate eczema. The solution? Take it in supplement form. Symptoms should improve gradually, and you'll very likely see a decreased need to use antihistamines.

Bugs that Make You Well

Now for the bugs. *Probiotics* is the name for a general class of "good" bacteria that are essential for proper digestive system function. If digestion isn't working properly, the body is more prone to allergies and skin disturbances.

A 2007 Swedish study published in the *American Journal of Allergy and Clinical Immunology* reported that probiotic-supplemented children of mothers with allergies experienced significant reductions in eczema. "Treated infants had less ... eczema at two years of age and therefore possibly run a reduced risk to develop later respiratory allergic disease," wrote lead researcher Thomas Abrahamsson from Linkoping University Hospital. And that research is in line with a previous study from Finland that reported that children who received a particular kind of probiotic—the Lactobacillus rhamnosus GG bacteria—were a whopping 40 percent less likely to develop atopic eczema at four years of age than children who received a placebo.

Probiotic supplementation is especially critical if a lot of yeast is present, and will help restore a healthy balance of microbes in the digestive tract. Since a healthy digestive tract is critical for prevention of allergies, working with a health-care provider who can eliminate yeast and replenish some of the good bacteria through probiotics use will help to diminish eczema flare-ups.

Natural Prescription for Eczema

Gamma linolenic acid or GLA (found in evening primrose oil, borage oil, and black currant oil): Start with 2 g of evening primrose oil and work up to 6 g. Each gram of evening primrose oil contains about 100 mg of GLA. (Alternately, you can take straight GLA, available as a supplement on my website, www.jonnybowden.com.) Use for at least four weeks. Balance with 1 g of omega-3 fish oils.

Probiotics: At least 10 billion bacteria

Food allergy testing: IgG allergy tests are best. (Many doctors who practice integrative or complementary medicine will perform these.)

Zinc: 25 mg

Selenium: 200 mcg

Chamomile: A natural anti-itch treatment. Boil up tea and pat on affected areas with cotton. (Let the tea cool first, lest you replace itching with burning.)

Witch hazel: A soothing anti-itch remedy. Apply on eczema as needed.

Colloidal oatmeal bath: Lukewarm, before bed, whenever necessary.

Note: All dosages are daily and come in pill or capsule form unless otherwise noted.

Emotional Pain

Ease Your Symptoms with Emotional Freedom Technique

IF YOU'RE IN EMOTIONAL PAIN and distress, one natural treatment you should definitely check out is emotional freedom technique, or EFT.

Described by its founder, Gary Craig, as an emotional version of acupuncture, EFT is a non-invasive treatment that people use to liberate themselves from the energy blocks caused by anger, grief, negative self-image, self-defeating beliefs, and even disease.

Candace Pert, Ph.D., author of the groundbreaking book *Molecules of Emotion*, says that "EFT is at the forefront of the new healing movement," and Deepak Chopra has said "EFT offers great healing benefits."

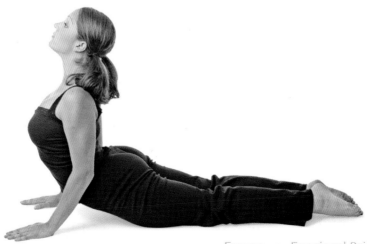

The premise of EFT is based on the idea that there are energy pathways throughout the body (similar to the meridians in acupuncture) and that if this energy is not flowing well, health is negatively affected. Acupuncture stimulates these meridians with needles but in EFT you stimulate these energy pathways with fingertips. Specifically, you simply tap with the fingertips on nine specific spots while stating an affirmation related to the issue you want to address (more on that in a moment).

Tapping Pain Away

There are nine "tapping points" on the body, one located on the top of the head, five located on various parts of the face and chin, two on the body, and one on the wrists. It doesn't matter in what order you tap them, just so long as you hit them all (though it makes it a snap to remember if you go from top to bottom). The classic technique taught by founder Gary Craig relies on using just two fingers of one hand for the tapping, but other versions uses four fingers of both hands.

WORTH KNOWING

There are many excellent video tutorials on how to do EFT, most of them free. Try Googling "tutorial on how to do EFT" or search for them on YouTube.

"There are a number of acupuncture meridians on your fingertips, and when you tap with your fingertips you are likely using not only the meridians you are tapping on, but also the ones on your fingers," he says.

The affirmations that you say while tapping have to do with creating a sense of self-acceptance that includes accepting the issue you are addressing. So, for example, if you're addressing migraine headaches, you might say something like, "Even though I have this blinding headache, I deeply and completely accept myself." (It doesn't seem to matter whether you believe the affirmation or not. What's important is that you say it anyway.) You repeat the statement, tuning in to "the problem" while tapping the meridians. It's that simple.

The idea is that thinking about the problem while doing the tapping, i.e., "tuning in," will bring about the very energy disruptions involved in the problem. (You know this is true for yourself if you've ever started thinking about an anxiety-producing situation in your life and noticed your heart racing, even though you didn't get off the couch. Thoughts have power.) The tapping and the affirmation create a correction that will then balance the disrupted energy.

Curing the Incurable

EFT falls squarely into the camp of what might be called "energy medicine" or "energy healing."

"The body will tend to heal itself if its energy is allowed to flow," says urologist Eric Robins, M.D., a huge EFT proponent. "The biggest thing that blocks that flow of energy is how emotional issues and past traumas are held in the body."

Whether the positive results that people report from EFT are due to the actual tapping of the meridians, the focus on acceptance, or some unspecified neurobiological change that may ensue when performing the tapping is hard to say. What's pretty clear is that there is a huge emotional component to most physical problems, and the power of neurochemicals in the brain is nearly as great as that of any pharmacy.

I don't know whether those neurochemicals can heal every disease on earth—or even all the conditions that EFT proponents claim to be able to improve. What I do know is that it has dramatic results for many people. Even the *Wall Street Journal*, in a 2007 article called "The Unmedicated Mind," quoted people who had tried EFT and found relief that they had been unable to get through conventional routes.

"It's possible to clear emotional issues at a deep enough level that physical healing results," says Robins. "I see EFT 'cure' things that are incurable all the time."

Gout

Snack on Cherries to Reduce Pain and Inflammation

GOUT, ALSO KNOWN AS metabolic arthritis, is a painful, largely inherited disorder in which the body can't properly metabolize uric acid. Usually the bloodstream contains a small amount of the stuff, but in gout there's a lot of it. The body doesn't know what to do with the excess so it bunches it up into nasty little crystals that get deposited in areas like the big toe and the joints, causing a lot of pain and discomfort.

Nutritionally minded health-care professionals and other healers have known for eons that cherries help relieve the pain of gout, but now we have a scientific explanation for why. Compounds in cherries lower levels of uric acid in the blood. Less uric acid, fewer disposal problems, fewer crystals, less pain. A study at the University of California–Davis showed that consuming two servings' worth of cherries daily (280 g total) after an overnight fast significantly lowered the blood uric acid of women by as much as 15 percent. And in another study, volunteers' blood levels of uric acid decreased significantly up to five hours after a breakfast meal of forty-five fresh, pitted Bing cherries.

The Power of Red: The Miracle of Anthocyanins

The secret to the benefits of cherries and cherry juice are compounds called *anthocyanins*. These are the particular pigments in cherries that give them their bright red color and are considered to be the key to helping the body relieve inflammation. It's believed that the anthocyanins in the cherries cause the decrease in uric acid and the relief from the pain of gout.

You've undoubtedly heard of a class of medicinal pain relievers called "Cox 2 inhibitors," drugs that include Celebrex (and used to include Vioxx and Bextra, but both were withdrawn from the market because the increased the risk of heart disease and stroke.) COX stands for *cyclooxygenase*, which is produced in the body in two major flavors, COX-1 and COX-2. It's COX-2 that is responsible for signaling pain and inflammation. The various over-the-counter NSAIDS (like Advil and Motrin) block both COX 1 and COX-2 as does aspirin—but the problem is that COX-1 has some valuable uses so you really don't want to block it. The COX-2 inhibitor drugs inhibited the pain-signaling COX-2 molecules without touching the non-inflammatory COX-1s.

Unfortunately there were some serious side effects with those drugs, which is why two of them were taken off the market. But anthocyanins, which are natural COX-2 inhibitors, produce a similar effect with none of the side effects.

Cherries (and raspberries) have the highest yields of pure anthocyanins. In one study, the COX inhibitory activity of anthocyanins from cherries was comparable to those of ibuprofen and naproxen. And researchers feel

WORTH KNOWING

Cherry juice is another way to get the gout-relieving benefits of cherries. In my book *The 150 Healthiest Foods on Earth*, I shared one of my favorite desserts: frozen cherries. (You can get them in almost any grocery.) I take them directly from the freezer, put them in a bowl, and mix them with raw milk or yogurt, which promptly freezes on the cold cherries, forming a kind of cherry-flavored sherbet. Top with slivered almonds and enjoy!

that in addition to helping with pain and inflammation, anthocyanins may help lower heart attack and stroke risk if consumed on a regular basis. As a bonus, these same anthocyanins may significantly reduce your risk for colon cancer, the third leading cancer in the United States.

A Dietary Connection to Gout that Will Surprise You

For years we've thought that gout was a disease brought on by an overly rich, fatty diet (hence it's nickname as "the rich man's disease"). But a study in the *British Medical Journal* followed more than 46,000 men with no previous history of gout for 12 years, compiling copious research on what they ate and drank. What they found was a direct relationship between the intake of sugar sweetened soft drinks and the risk of gout. Compared to men who consumed less than one serving of soft drinks a month, those consuming five to six sodas a week significantly raised their risk of gout by 29 percent. Even worse, those who consumed just two sodas a day increased their risk by an incredible 85 percent!

Natural Prescription for Gout

Dietary: No sodas, sweetened fruit juices, or other sugared beverages. Reduce sugar and especially fructose in general. Eat cherries or drink cherry juice as often as possible.

Heart Disease

Strengthen and Protect Your Heart with This Array of Natural Aids

L-carnitine

D-ribose

CoQ10

Magnesium

HERE'S A STORY I'll never forget. My mother was admitted to the hospital in the last week of her eighty-seven-year life, which up to then had been extremely healthy and pretty happy. The doctors diagnosed her with congestive heart failure. I immediately asked that, in addition to whatever treatment the doctors prescribed, she be put on a high dose of coenzyme Q10 (CoQ10).

The first doctor told me he didn't know what that was. The second doctor said he had heard of it but it couldn't do any good and wasn't on their hospital pharmacy list. And the head nurse said, "Oh, that's some kind of enzyme that the heart makes when it's in trouble, right?" I knew right there we were in for trouble.

It didn't matter that I faxed them fifty pages of peer-reviewed literature from the National Institute of Medicine. They wouldn't budge. And my mother, bless her heart, was of the generation that believed that if the doctor told you something, that was it. You didn't question it.

Let me be blunt: The doctors who told me that they didn't know what CoQ10 was or that it couldn't possibly help were idiots. "Although coenzyme Q10 represents one of the greatest breakthroughs for the treatment of cardio-vascular disease as well as for other diseases, the resistance of the medical profession to using this essential nutrient represents one of the greatest potential tragedies in medicine," says my friend, board-certified cardiologist, nutritionist, and noted author Stephen Sinatra, M.D.

So What Is CoQ10, Anyway?

CoQ10 has been an approved drug in Japan for congestive heart failure since 1974. And several studies have demonstrated a relationship between depleted CoQ10 levels and heart disease.

CoQ10 isn't a vitamin; it actually belongs to a family called *ubiquinones*, and it's found in most tissues in the body. It's essential for the manufacture of the body's energy molecule, adenosine triphosphate, or ATP. Virtually every one of the studies investigating the effect of CoQ10 on heart muscle function has reported significant and positive results.

"If there is just one thing you do to help maintain your heart's health," says Sinatra, "make sure you're taking CoQ10 daily."

L-Carnitine: Energy for a Weak Heart

L- carnitine is a vitamin-like compound that you can obtain from your diet, but it's also made in the body. The best way to think of it is as a shuttle bus. Its job is to escort fatty acids into the mitochondria (energy centers) of the cells where they can be "burned" for energy. Because the heart gets 60 percent of its energy from fat, it's critically important that the body have enough L-carnitine to "shuttle" the fatty acids into the muscle cells of the heart.

The strongest research evidence for the benefit of L-carnitine supplementation comes from studies of patients being treated for various forms of cardiovascular disease. People who take L-carnitine supplements soon after suffering a heart attack may be less likely to suffer a subsequent heart attack, die of heart disease, experience chest pain and abnormal heart rhythms, or develop congestive heart failure (a condition in which the heart loses its ability to pump blood effectively). A well-designed study of seventy heart-failure patients found that three-year survival was significantly higher in the group receiving 2 g a day of L-carnitine compared to the group receiving a placebo.

Carnitine also appears to improve exercise capacity in people with coronary artery disease. In one study, the walking capacity of patients with intermittent claudication—a painful cramping sensation in the muscles of the legs due to decreased oxygen supply—improved significantly when they were given oral L-carnitine. In another study, patients with peripheral arterial disease of the legs were able to increase their walking distance by 98 meters when supplemented with carnitine, almost twice what those given a placebo were able to do. Congestive heart failure patients have experienced an increase in exercise endurance on only 900 mg of carnitine per day. It also appears to help alleviate the symptoms of angina.

Nutritionists have long used the combination of L-carnitine and CoQ10 as an "energy" cocktail. Though it doesn't necessarily make you feel more "get up and go" (although for many people it does just that!), it definitely helps give your heart muscle the tools it needs to function optimally. If you think of your body as an automobile, then L-carnitine and CoQ10 can be thought of as agents (like spark plugs) that help turn the gas in the tank into energy to make the car go.

D-Ribose: A Mighty Molecule

D-ribose, the third component of this quartet (which Sinatra nicknamed the "Awesome Foursome"), can be thought of as the actual gas. D-ribose is a five-carbon sugar that seems to accelerate the recovery of energy during and following cardiac ischemia, a condition in which blood flow to the heart muscle is obstructed. One of Sinatra's coauthors, James Roberts, M.D., is a marathoner who began using D-ribose on himself and found that taking it before and after a run eliminated many of the problems, like pain, soreness, stiffness, and fatigue, associated with long-distance runs. He began putting his patients on D-ribose and found that his sickest patients improved within days.

"Giving D-ribose to patients both before (as a cardioprotective) and following (to restore lost energy) cardiac intervention has proven to be an effective way to improve clinical outcome," says Sinatra.

D-ribose is made in the cells, and the body uses it in a variety of ways that are all critical to cellular function. When blood flow and oxygen are compromised as in, for example, ischemia, hearts can lose a lot of their stores of ATP (the energy molecule), and it can take up to ten days to normalize cardiac function. When you give D-ribose to patients with ischemia, energy recovery and function can return to normal in an average of one to two days, according to Sinatra.

Any time the energy reserves of the muscle are depleted, whether through exercise or a heart condition, ribose supplementation can help. "An adequate dose of ribose will usually result in symptom improvement very quickly," says Sinatra. "Remember that ribose therapy directly supports the heart's ability to preserve and rebuild its energy pool," he says.

The Perfect Quartet

Vegetarians often lack L-carnitine in their diets (and most certainly lack D-ribose, which is primarily found in red meat and veal). Carnitine (carnis means "meat" or "flesh") is found in mutton, lamb, beef, red meat, and pork and in only tiny amounts in plant foods.

Though certain vegetables, meats, and fish contain CoQ10, we only consume a tiny amount in our diet, not nearly enough to have a clinically important benefit. Many people feel a lot better on an "energy" cocktail of L-carnitine and CoQ10.

Rounding out the quartet with D-ribose and magnesium, as suggested by Sinatra, is a great idea, especially for heart patients. (Magnesium helps because it is critical for the making of ATP, has an important effect on cellular metabolism, has been found helpful in a wide range of cardiac conditions, and because approximately three-fourths of the population are deficient in it!)

When you consume magnesium in optimal amounts it improves myriad heart conditions, including angina, arrhythmia, cardiomyopathy, mitral valve prolapse, intermittent claudication, and low HDL (the "good" cholesterol). It improves energy production within the heart, dilating the arteries and help-ing blood do its job of delivering oxygen to the heart more effectively. Studies have shown that people dying of a heart attack have lower magnesium levels than people of the same age dying from other causes.

There's an interesting circular relationship between stress and magnesium. Stress causes low magnesium levels, low magnesium levels cause stress, and the circle continues downward. Both stress and magnesium deficiency set you up for cardiovascular disease. In animal studies, giving animals magnesium has been shown to prevent this process from happening, protecting heart tissue from destruction.

Let me be perfectly clear: The combination of CoQ10, L-carnitine, D-ribose, and magnesium doesn't "cure" heart disease. But to not use it as part of a treatment protocol to strengthen and protect the heart would be a huge mistake.

How Omega-3s Help the Heart

Omega-3 blood levels are one of the best predictors of sudden heart attack. Those with the highest risk for heart attacks have the lowest levels of omega-3s. In Britain, heart attack survivors are now prescribed fish oil supplements for life in keeping with the guidelines of the British National Institute for Health and Clinical Excellence. Many physicians also consider supplementa-tion with omega-3 fatty acids an important part of nutritional treatment for diabetes and metabolic syndrome.

There's also the fact that omega-3s (fish oil) have a strong impact on one of the most important risk factors for heart disease—high triglycerides. Fish oil supplements reduce triglyceride levels by up to 40 percent in some research, an astonishingly high amount. The Agency for Healthcare Research and Quality (the research arm of the U.S. Department of Health and Human Services) analyzed 123 studies on omega-3 fatty acids and concluded that "omega-3 fatty acids demonstrated a consistently large, significant effect on triglycerides—a net decrease of 10 to 33 percent." The effect is most pronounced in those with high triglycerides to begin with. Even the extremely conservative American Heart Association recommends 2 to 4 g of the two omega-3 fats found in fish oil (EPA and DHA) for patients who need to lower triglycerides.

WORTH KNOWING

Just as we were going to press, my friend and go-to guy for all things related to fibromyalgia and chronic fatigue syndrome, Jacob Teitelbaum, M.D., wrote to tell me of a just-published study showing that in chronic fatigue and fibromyalgia patients, ribose increased energy an average of 45 percent.

"It is even more incredible in heart disease," he said. Teitelbaum told me that he suspects ribose "will be the most important nutritional discovery of the decade." According to Teitelbaum, dosing is critical. He recommends 5 grams three times a day for 3 to 6 weeks, then twice a day. "This is too important of a nutrient discovery to be missed," he says.

Read about the story at www.ncbi.nlm.nih.gov/pubmed/17109576.

Another major risk factor for heart disease is hypertension, or high blood pressure. Fish oil lowers blood pressure, albeit modestly. But its effect on cardiovascular disease overall is anything but modest. Study after study has shown that the omega-3 fatty acids found in fish reduce the risk of death, heart attack, stroke, and abnormal heart rhythms (arrhythmias). It's been estimated that proper omega-3 fatty acid intake could reduce the rate of fatal arrhythmias by 30 percent. More than 70,000 lives could be saved each year if Americans had sufficient omega-3s in their bodies, estimates Harvard's Andrew Stoll, M.D., author of *The Omega-3 Connection*.

One More Benefit

Another one of the many benefits of omega-3s is that they are anti-inflammatory. The full importance of inflammation as a factor in disease is only just now beginning to be fully appreciated.

Since inflammation is a component of every major degenerative disease from heart disease to Alzheimer's, the importance of foods and supplements that are anti-inflammatory can't be overstated. The anti-inflammatory action of the omega-3 fats found in fish oil has been proven in dozens of research studies, including the ongoing ATTICA study in Athens, Greece, that demonstrated direct evidence showing that omega-3s reduce blood markers of inflammation like C-reactive protein, which are increasingly accepted as key risk factors for heart disease. The anti-inflammatory action of fish oil makes it a terrific supplement for arthritis, for aging and aching joints, and for the inflamed airways of those suffering with asthma.

Stress and Cardiovascular Health

Too much stress causes magnesium to be depleted, which can lead to hypertension, coronary artery constriction, arrhythmias, and heart attack. Here's how it works: When you're under too much stress your body overproduces substances called catecholamines. While some act as neurotransmitters and make us feel good (dopamine), catecholamines also act as hormones in the blood, and too high a level of them will cause magnesium to be released from cells into the blood and then excreted in urine.

A low magnesium level in the cells causes heart tissue destruction. End result: heart attack.

The Magical Pomegranate

Pomegranate juice may just turn out to be one of the great natural weapons against heart disease. A daily dose of this delicious juice may go a long way toward keeping you from becoming a statistic. Studies in Israel have shown that, taken daily, pomegranate juice prevented the thickening of arteries. It also slowed down the oxidation of cholesterol by almost half—which to me is more impressive than just reducing cholesterol, since cholesterol is only a problem in the body when it's oxidized. And it makes sense that pomegranate juice would have that effect because of its stunning antioxidant content.

"Pomegranate juice contains the highest antioxidant capacity compared to other juices, red wine, and green tea," says Michael Aviram, D.Sc., a professor of biochemistry and medicine at the Rappaport Family Institute for Research in the Medical Sciences in Haifa, Israel, who led the team of Israeli researchers.

The research on pomegranate juice is mounting, and it's impressive. In one study, published in the *American Journal of Cardiology*, forty-five participants—all of whom had some form of ischemic heart disease—were divided into two groups. For three months, one group received 8 1/2 ounces of pomegranate juice daily while the other group got a placebo drink with the same number of calories, coloring, and flavor. The researchers found that blood flow to the heart improved by about 17 percent in the pomegranate group while declining about 18 percent in the placebo group. And this benefit was realized without any negative effects whatsoever.

Natural Prescription for Heart Health

Coenzyme Q10: 100 to 300 mg

L-carnitine: 500 to 4,000 mg

D-ribose: 5 g

Magnesium: 400 to 800 mg

FOR ADDED EFFECTIVENESS:

Multivitamin

Fish oil: 2 g

Vitamin E from mixed tocopherols or gamma-tocopherol: 400 IU

Taurine: 1 to 3 g

Pomegranate Juice: 4 to 8 ounces daily or as often as possible

Note: All dosages are daily dosages and in pill or capsule form unless otherwise noted.

Yogurt

Heartburn

Calm the Fires with Enzymes and Bugs

MORE THAN 50 million
Americans experience heartburn

Probiotics HCl

at least twice a week, and about 25 million on a
daily basis.

For almost a hundred years, many of us have relied on antacids to quench the flames of fire in the belly, and products such as Tums, Tagamet, Maalox, and Mylanta produce annual sales of more than a $1 billion. When those aren't enough, we turn to prescription drugs that block the production of stomach acid even longer than their over-the-counter cousins. Prevacid and Nexium are among the five top-selling prescription drugs in the U.S., and heartburn drugs are now among the most widely prescribed medications in the country, producing more than $13 billion in sales in 2004.

But consistently taking acid suppressors like heartburn drugs over time as a way of managing symptoms is a horrendous idea. (Don't kill the messenger here.) Fortunately, there are other, better (and healthier) options. Keep reading.

Heartburn, Indigestion, and Reflux Explained

Heartburn is actually not associated with the heart at all but was labeled and named "heartburn" because it can feel like a heart attack. For some, that burning sensation can become unbearable.

The terms heartburn and indigestion are often used interchangeably, but there is a clear distinction between the two. Though they both have similar triggers, and treatment may be the same in many instances, indigestion isn't the same thing as heartburn. Indigestion is, in fact, a *condition*. It is a feeling of discomfort and pain in the upper abdomen and chest and may also be accompanied by a feeling of fullness, bloating, and belching.

Heartburn, which is described as a burning sensation in the chest and stomach, is a *symptom* of indigestion. The burning sensation may even travel up toward the neck. It's also a symptom of another common condition called gastrointestinal reflux disease, (GERD), or acid reflux. In addition to heartburn, symptoms of acid reflux may include persistent sore throat, hoarseness, chronic cough, asthma, heart-like chest pain, and a feeling of a lump in the throat.

The Role of Acid

So it might seem like an open and shut case. Hydrochloric acid "causes" heartburn—knock out the hydrochloric acid production with a pill, symptom gone, case closed. Right?

No.

"The myth that underlies the conventional treatment of 'acid indigestion,' and the implied message in all these commercials, is that heartburn happens because we've got too much acid in our stomachs," writes integrative medicine icon Jonathan Wright, M.D. Wright has been in the forefront of the movement to educate people about the overwhelming importance of hydrochloric acid in human health—he even wrote a book about it called *Why Stomach Acid is Good for You* (highly recommended).

Here's why suppressing acid is such a bad idea: Hydrochloric acid (HCl) is responsible for activating enzymes in the stomach that then allow us to break down the proteins that we've eaten. With limited HCl, those enzymes are not activated and the proteins are not broken down. Result? Badly impaired digestion. Stomach acid stays in the stomach and builds up, so we end up with more acid in our stomach that can potentially reflux back up into the esophagus.

Low HCl is a major factor in many digestive disorders. Wright believes that diseases as disparate as rheumatoid arthritis, childhood asthma, osteoporosis, chronic fatigue, and depression all have in common low stomach acid. Childhood asthma is a good case in point: More than 80 percent of children diagnosed with asthma have exhibited low HCl levels. In fact, according to Wright, hydrochloric acid can be a significant part of the cure for children with asthma. "In hundreds of cases," he says, "I have found that more than 50 percent of children who come to me with asthma can have their wheezing cured by simply normalizing their stomach acid and properly administering vitamin B12, with no bronchodilators and no corticosteroids."

Bacteria Thrive in a Non-Acidic Environment

Most bacteria can't survive an acidic environment, so killing off acid production creates nirvana for bacteria. Without acid to kill them off, they have a party and reproduce like rabbits. Bacterial overgrowth in the stomach and small intestine can lead to a host of symptoms, including gas, constipation, diarrhea, and even infections. Overgrowth of bacteria can also interfere with the absorption of vitamin B12 and can interfere with the proper digestion and absorption of fats and sugars. And low acid can contribute to food allergies. Why? Because if we don't have enough acid in our stomachs to digest food, we can't adequately break down foods, and we develop what's called a leaky gut. With a leaky gut, incompletely digested food particles escape back into our system. Our immune cells go "Hey, what's this? We don't recognize these dudes," and then proceed to attack what they perceive as "foreign invaders." This can easily be the birth of a food allergy.

Maybe you figure, okay, acid does all these good things for me, but it's still giving me serious heartburn. Don't I need to get rid of it for that reason alone? If you think this way, you're hardly alone. Most people think the way to get rid of acid reflux is to simply get rid of the acid. (Pharmaceutical companies and those making $13 billion a year from the sale of antacids are counting on you thinking this way.) If you're one of the many, many people who think an antacid is the answer to your acid problem, I hope you'll reconsider after reading this section.

What's Wrong with Acid Suppression? A Lot

The problem isn't that there's too much acid—in fact, it's sometimes the opposite (read on). The problem is that the acid sometimes goes to the wrong place, flowing back—or "refluxing"—into our esophagus where it can really burn the delicate tissues. This reflex reaction may in part be due to a muscle in the lower part of the esophagus (called the LES, or lower esophageal sphincter) that is weakened or stops working correctly. As long as the LES stays closed like it's supposed to, you're good to go. No heartburn symptoms, no burning.

"Given the right environment and enough time to heal itself, an irritated or injured LES often returns to its normal, healthy state, eliminating heartburn. Even the more severe condition of GERD can often [but not always] be brought under control by this approach to treatment," Wright says.

And here's the kicker: Heartburn can also occur—in fact, it frequently does occur—when hydrochloric acid levels in the stomach are too low! According to Wright, the overwhelming majority of people with indigestion have a stomach acid deficiency. Keep in mind that a healthy gut and optimal digestion depend on adequate acid in the stomach. After all, acid promotes the digestion and utilization of critical nutrients and amino acids, not to mention vitamin B12, folic acid, and calcium. If there isn't enough acid to trigger the activation of the important digestive enzyme pepsin, you're out of luck. Your digestion is impaired and with it, your body's ability to extract healing nutrients from your food.

If you're still not convinced that the problem isn't too much acid, consider this: The incidence of heartburn and GERD increases as you get older. But as we age, we produce less hydrochloric acid, not more. (The elderly have the least HCl of all.)

"If too much acid were causing these problems, teenagers should have frequent heartburn while grandma and grandpa should have much less," notes Wright. Of course we know that just the opposite is true.

So while it may bring temporary symptom relief, acid suppression isn't the answer. A far better way to permanently cure heartburn and indigestion is to improve the digestive process and heal the lower esophageal sphincter so it works properly. With a few changes in your diet and with the use of safe, effective supplements like those in the natural prescription I'm going to tell you about, you can restore healthy digestion, heal the gut, and produce improvement in a wide variety of symptoms and health conditions.

By creating a healthy gut environment, which includes a healthy amount of stomach acid, and not triggering inappropriate behavior on the part of the LES (usually by simply eliminating foods that do just that), you are well on the way to banning heartburn symptoms from your life.

Step One: It Starts with Food

The first thing you want to do is eliminate known triggers that cause the LES to pop open inappropriately (allowing any amount of acid, even a little, to bounce back into the esophagus).

Off the food list comes caffeine, including caffeinated soft drinks, tea, and chocolate—all of which are known for relaxing the LES, allowing stomach contents to reflux back up into the esophagus. Chocolate contains concentrations of *theobromine*, a compound that occurs naturally in many plants, such as those that produce cocoa, tea, and coffee, and which is known for relaxing the LES. Other foods that also relax or weaken the LES are tomatoes, spicy foods, onions, citrus fruits and juices, alcohol, and tobacco.

And then there are foods that slow down digestion, keeping the food in your stomach longer. This can result in increased pressure in the stomach, which in turn puts more pressure on a weakened LES, allowing reflux of stomach contents. These include fried or fatty foods and large meals.

Many people try drinking milk to ease heartburn before sleep, but milk may end up causing more heartburn distress. Drinking milk and eating a big meal at dinner can be a recipe for disaster. It's a myth that milk can "coat" the stomach or help heartburn. On the contrary, it can aggravate the heck out of it. And the higher the fat content in the milk, the worse it can be.

Here's one thing you can have: water, pure and clean (I know it's not the most exciting thing in the world, but it works). Some researchers theorize that heartburn is a sign of an internal water shortage, especially dehydration in the upper part of the GI tract. So try drinking up first before you overload your system with antacids and medications, but do this in-between, not during, meals: You'll want to drink only about 4 ounces of water with a meal so that you don't further dilute HCl, which will be needed to digest incoming proteins.

Step Two: On to Enzymes and Probiotics

The natural cure for heartburn is a two-step process. First, get the food triggers under control (see above). Then add the "big guns": digestive enzymes and probiotics.

Digestive enzymes are made in your body naturally (and turned on in the presence of stomach acid), but many of us make less of them as we get older. Fortunately, they can be taken as a supplement, and there are many terrific formulas on the market (check my website, www.jonnybowden.com, for ones I recommend). Digestive enzymes have been shown to be extremely beneficial in the treatment of heartburn. Also called bitters, they've been around for centuries in the form of plants and herbs.

Gentian root is one well-known bitter. Gentian improves digestion by increasing appetite and stimulating digestive juices and pancreatic activity. It also stimulates the secretion of hydrochloric acid and bile and is known for relieving gallbladder problems and indigestion. Most supplements these days contain a mix of enzymes like bromelain, found in pineapple, papain from papaya, and proteolytic enzymes, which are animal-derived enzymes that break down proteins.

I recommend a digestive enzyme supplement that also contains HCl; many good supplements do. Alternately you can take an HCl supplement alone. The most common form of HCl supplement is called betaine-HCl. Betaine-HCl is a combination of betaine—a product derived from sugar beets—and hydrochloric acid. (Note: Plain betaine is also known as trimethylglycine, or TMG, the chemical name for betaine. Don't confuse the two. Betaine, or TMG, is a valuable supplement used to bring down the body's levels of an inflammatory compound found in the blood called homocysteine. But it has nothing to do with digestion. For that you need betaine bound to hydrochloric acid, i.e., Betaine-HCl.)

Probiotics, also known as "good bacteria," are wonderful for promoting healthy digestion. In fact, they're essential for it. Remember, your gut is a garden balanced between the "good" bacteria (the flowers) and the "bad" (the weeds). Everyone has some of both—the trick is to keep them in balance. The "good" bacteria—probiotics—are beneficial bacteria, such as Lacto-bacillus acidophilus and Bifidobacterium bifidum. Probiotic bacteria favorably alter the intestinal microflora balance, inhibit the growth of harmful bacteria (like Candida albicans, or "yeast"), promote good digestion, boost immune function, and increase resistance to infection. Probiotics also contain enzymes to help break down and digest dairy products like lactose in milk.

The best place to find probiotics is in yogurts that contain active cultures. But you can also increase the content by purchasing a high-quality probiotic formula. (I have several excellent ones listed on my website.) Take the probiotics as a pill or buy in powder form and stir it into water or yogurt.

This Just In

Just as this manuscript was being completed, I received an email that my good friend, the great integrative medicine guru Leo Galland, M.D., was appearing on the Today show. Galland went on national television to speak about virtually everything we've discussed in this section—why you need stomach acid to be at the top of the list, and why acid-lowering drugs are a really bad idea. You can see his Today show appearance online at www.fatresistancediet.com.

Natural Prescription for Heartburn

Digestive enzymes or digestive enzymes with hydrochloric acid: (take with every meal, dose dependent on improvement)

Note: if you have an ulcer, work with a health professional. Don't self-treat.

Probiotics: 10 billion. Keep refrigerated. (Note: Probiotics are available in either pill form or as a powdered supplement that can be mixed in water.)

Optional: Deglycyrrhizinated licorice: 380 mg or 1 to 2 tablets chewed and swallowed on an empty stomach, three to four times a day as needed

Diet: Avoid refined sugar, caffeine, alcohol, and citrus fruits. Eat slowly and chew well. Eat yogurt and drink water.

Smoking: Stop.

Note: The above dosages are daily and in pill or capsule form unless otherwise specified.

Hepatitis C
Try This Powerful Combo Cure

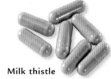

N-acetyl-cysteine

HEPATITIS C is a disease in which many outcomes are possible. I believe fervently that what you do and the choices you make can have a profound influence on the course the disease takes.

Milk thistle

Let's get this out of the way right off the bat: The single best thing you can do if you've got hepatitis C or any liver disease is to stop drinking. Completely. No kidding. Alcohol puts a strain on your liver, which is not so bad if your liver is healthy but is lethal if it's not. So if you've got hepatits C, whatever else you do, you need to stop drinking.

Alpha lipoic acid

Selenium

A Medical Hero Takes on the Establishment

I first learned about the natural cure I'm going to tell you about from Burt Berkson. I'll introduce him so you'll understand why I paid as much attention as I did to his recommendation, and why I'm going to pass it on to you with a ringing, unqualified endorsement. I consider Burt Berkson a medical hero.

Years ago, Berkson was doing his internship at a hospital in Cleveland when two people were brought in by ambulance in pretty dire condition. They had been hiking, had eaten some highly poisonous mushrooms, and were close to death. Berkson remembered reading some research on a substance called alpha lipoic acid (ALA), which, in addition to being great for managing blood sugar, was an amazing free-radical scavenger. He appealed to the hospital to let him try ALA on the couple, but was turned down since no one had ever heard of it and it wasn't in the hospital's pharmacy. He was basically told there was nothing that could be done for the couple and if there was, the powers that be at the hospital would certainly have known about it. What did a mere intern think he could do with some nutritional supplement no one had ever heard of? And besides, what could an intern know that a resident or attending physician didn't?

Well, quite a lot actually.

Berkson, who is not only an M.D. but just happens to have a Ph.D. in microbiology with an advanced specialty in mushroom toxology, knew a bit about liver disease. Risking censure and loss of his internship, he called an old colleague, Fred Bartter at the National Institutes of Health, who arranged to fly in some ALA. He administered it to the dying couple.

And they're alive and well today.

That, by the way, is medical courage.

So when Burt Berkson talks about the liver, I listen.

Back in 1999, Berkson published a paper called *A conservative triple antioxidant approach to the treatment of hepatitis C: A combination of alpha lipoic acid (thioctic acid), silymarin, and selenium: Three case histories*. In it, he suggested a basic protocol of three supplements that would protect the liver from free-radical damage, increase the levels of other fundamental antioxidants, and interfere with viral proliferation.

That protocol is the core of the "natural cure" for hepatitis C. I believe every single person with hepatitis C or liver disease of any kind should be on it.

Helping the Liver

You can support the liver in four major ways:

1. **Don't add to its burden.** I know I said it earlier but it bears repeating: number one on the list of the liver's biggest burdens is alcohol, so stop drinking. Immediately. No kidding. And stop taking acetaminophen (found in Tylenol and other medications). Acetaminophen poisoning is the number-one cause of hospital admissions for liver failure in the United States. Think what people who drink and then take Tylenol for a hangover are doing to their poor liver. Though many establishment medical types will tell you acetaminophen is "safe" in reasonable doses, I'm a hardliner on acetaminophen: If you have—or suspect you have—liver problems, the only safe dose of acetaminophen is zero.

2. **Do a periodic detoxification.** There are dozens of ways to do this, using just raw foods, lightly steamed vegetables, broths, fresh vegetable juice, medical foods like Metagenics Ultra-Clear, or any combination thereof. Many excellent books give details. One of my favorites is *The New Detox Diet* by my friend, Elson Haas, M.D.

3. **Eat a liver-friendly diet.** Obviously, the fewer chemicals, preservatives, and artificial ingredients the liver has to get rid of, the better. Some foods are particularly liver friendly. Turmeric, the spice that makes Indian food yellow, contains natural anti-inflammatory *curcuminoids*, has anticancer activity, and is one of the best liver-friendly spices. Put it on everything. Wheatgrass juice and all the other "green drinks" that are high in chlorophyll are excellent. Coconut oil contains *lauric acid*, a well known

antimicrobial and antiviral fatty acid. Beets and beet juice have long had a reputation for being excellent for the liver, and in any case buying a juicer and making fresh vegetable juice on a daily basis (with some fruits thrown in if you like) is probably the best gift you can give your liver.

4. Take liver-friendly supplements. ALA is a powerful antioxidant that not only scavenges free radicals and helps protect cells but also helps regenerate vitamins C and E. It is one of the most powerful liver nutrients available. Berkson wrote a book about it called *The Alpha Lipoic Breakthrough*. Read it.

ALA also helps regenerate glutathione, arguably the body's most important antioxidant. Lester Packer, Ph.D., professor and senior researcher at the University of California for more than 40 years and author of *The Antioxidant Miracle*, has called ALA "probably the most potent naturally occurring antioxidant known to man."

By the time you read this, selenium's reputation will probably be even greater than it is today, and it's already held in pretty high esteem. This important mineral is a premier cancer fighter (it decreases the rate of prostate cancer) and in January 2007, one of the most conservative publications in medicine, *The Archives of Internal Medicine*, published an article showing that daily selenium supplements appear to suppress the progression of the viral load in patients with HIV infection. It's essential for those with hepatitis C. "Selenium acts as a birth control pill to the virus," Berkson told me.

The herb milk thistle (*silymarin*) is probably the premier liver nutrient. The active ingredient in milk thistle is silymarin, which is believed to be responsible for its medicinal qualities. Milk thistle has been used in Europe as a treatment for liver disease since the sixteenth century.

The Supporting Cast of Liver-Friendly Nutrients, Extracts, and Foods

There are a number of other important nutrients you should consider as part of a liver health/hep-C-fighting program.

N-A-C (N-acetyl-cysteine). This derivative of the amino acid L-cysteine is a precursor to the formation of the powerful antioxidant *glutathione*. It's one of the best ways to increase glutathione in the body (since glutathione isn't well absorbed orally, you have to make it). Recommended: 1,000 mg daily.

Whey protein powder. Though not technically a supplement, whey protein is another powerful way to increase the body's stores of glutathione and boost the immune system. Be sure to get a pure, high-quality powder made by a reputable company that markets to health professionals (there are several on my website, www.jonnybowden.com). You don't want one of the God-awful "fancy" protein shakes sweetened with sugar or some artificial chemical hazard that lines the shelves at the mall.

Vitamin C. This vitamin has antiviral activity, and intravenous vitamin C has long been used by practitioners of nutritional and integrative medicine for a variety of conditions. It has been championed for hepatitis by Robert Cathcart, M.D., a California physician who was recognized by the Society for Orthomolecular Health-Medicine as recipient of the Linus Pauling Award.

SAMe (S-adenosyl-methionine). SAMe is a naturally occurring molecule present in all living cells. It has many incredible benefits, (including a positive effect on depression and arthritis pain). For our purposes, it helps the liver to replenish important substances, notably the all-important glutathione. In one double-blind trial, people with cirrhosis of the liver due to alcoholism who took SAMe for two years had a 47 percent lower rate of death or need for liver transplantation compared with those who took a placebo.

Neominophagen. A component of licorice known as *glycyrrhizin* seems to have significant antiviral action. Neominophagen (also known as stronger neominophagen C or SNMC) is a kind of "superglycyrrhizin." It is widely used in Japan to treat hepatitis. Some cutting-edge practitioners in the United States have used it as well. It's injectable, so it has to be administered by a doctor.

Vitamin E. This vitamin has a place at the table in a liver-health protocol because of its antioxidant effects.

Artichokes. This vegetable has a long folk history in treating many liver diseases. Their active ingredient is *cynarin*, which has demonstrated liver-protecting effects. Artichoke extract is in a lot of liver-protection supplement formulas.

Dandelion root. Many people living healthily with hepatitis C swear by this herb and use it to make a tea.

Reishi and shiitake mushrooms. Chinese herbalists prize Reishi mushrooms for their protective effect on the liver. The bitterer the mushroom, the higher the level of *triterpenoids*, which give it its potency. It's usually made into a tea or taken as an extract.

Phosphatidylcholine. The active ingredient in the popular supplement lecithin is actually a substance called *phosphatidylcholine*. In animal research, it protects against cirrhosis and fibrosis. We know that choline—the prime constituent of phosphatidylcholine—is essential for normal liver function, and phos choline is an excellent "delivery system" for choline. In one double-blind

Natural Prescription for Hepatitis C

ESSENTIAL:

•**Alpha lipoic acid:** 900 to 1,200 mg

•**Selenium:** 200 to 400 mcg

•**Milk thistle (silymarin):** 900 mg

ALSO HIGHLY RECOMMENDED:

N-acetyl-cysteine: 1,000 mg

Whey protein powder: 1 to 2 servings

Dandelion tea: Frequently

Phosphatidylcholine: 3 g

Note: All dosages are daily dosages and in pill or capsule form unless otherwise noted.

study in England, chronic active hepatitis C patients were treated with 3 g of phos choline each day; they had significantly reduced symptoms compared to the control subjects. Many researchers have postulated that phosphatidylcholine has an ability to repair the membranes of liver cells.

You can die of old age with your hepatitis C (or even better, without it, if you're one of the lucky people who can clear it on your own). You don't have to die from it.

Herpes

Strike Back with Lysine

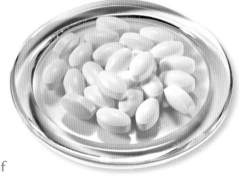

I DON'T KNOW ABOUT YOU, but when I was "coming up," as they say, herpes was the scourge of the sexual revolution.

AIDS was a few years away, and we were still way too naive to know about the dozens of other sexually transmitted diseases like Chlamydia or human papillomavirus. If you got herpes back then it was considered the death knell for your sex life. There were herpes support groups, for goodness' sake. (Remember, this was pre-Oprah.) Having herpes was the deepest, darkest secret you could possibly harbor.

Well, times have changed a lot, but herpes is still not something you'd put on your must-have list. Herpes simplex virus is a recurrent viral infection that causes outbreaks on any area of the body, particularly the mouth or genitals. (HSV-1 is the cold sore variety, HSV-2 the genital variety and yes, they can transfer back and forth. Sorry.)

More than 60 percent of those infected with herpes virus will have reoccurring outbreaks of herpes. While one person may only have one or two outbreaks per year, and some lucky folks have them only once every few years if that, others are plagued by this infectious, painful, sometimes dangerous, and always uncomfortable virus several times per month. Chicken pox, shingles, and cold sores—they're all part of the herpes family. And then, of course, there are those familiar outbreaks in the most unwanted of intimate places—always, it seems, just when you have the best chance of getting lucky.

Even if you've been fortunate enough never to have an outbreak of genital herpes, you've probably experienced a plain old garden-variety cold sore. And if you have, you've probably gone on the inevitable quest to find something—anything—that will make it go away: licorice root, homeopathic medicines, vitamin mega-doses, avoiding the sun, and any technique that reduces stress. They're all good and can help control an outbreak when it happens. But for true prevention you may want to consider some immune-enhancing strategies, and you might especially want to consider lysine.

Enter the Herpes Slayer

Lysine, an amino acid, has had a reputation as a first-line defense against herpes for a long time. Back in 1978, a multicenter study of lysine therapy in herpes simplex infection was published in the journal *Dermatologica*; the authors found that lysine "appears to suppress the clinical manifestations of the herpes virus." A number of studies followed over the years—one found that more patients were recurrence-free during lysine treatment (1,000 mg daily) while another found that 1,000 mg of lysine three times a day for six months resulted in fewer infections, less severe symptoms, and significantly less healing time.

In one other study, researchers surveyed 1,543 subjects with a questionnaire after a six-month trial period during which they took an average dose of 936 mg of lysine daily. The study included subjects with cold sores, canker sores, and genital herpes. Eighty-four percent of those surveyed said that lysine supplementation prevented recurrence or decreased the frequency of herpes infection. Whereas 79 percent described their symptoms as "severe" or "intolerable" without lysine, only 8 percent used these terms when taking lysine. Without lysine, 90 percent indicated that healing took six to fifteen days, but *with* lysine, 83 percent stated that lesions healed in five or fewer days. Overall, a stunning 88 percent of the people in the study considered supplemental lysine an effective form of treatment for herpes infection! Not bad for a nondrug intervention with no known side effects.

Lysine and Arginine

Lysine is considered an essential amino acid, defined as an amino acid that the body can't manufacture and therefore has to be obtained from food (or supplements). It works hand in hand with other essential amino acids to maintain growth, lean body mass, and the body's store of nitrogen, an essential part of all amino and nucleic acids, both of which are necessary to all life. But when it comes to herpes, lysine has a strange relationship with another (very important) amino acid, *arginine*.

Herpes is less likely to reproduce when the ratio of lysine to arginine favors lysine—when there's too much arginine and not enough lysine, the virus likes to replicate. Therefore, when you're fighting herpes, you want to make sure *not* to take arginine supplements, great as they may be for other things (like the heart and even sexual performance). Foods that have more lysine than arginine include fish, chicken, beef, lamb, milk, cheese, beans, brewer's yeast, mung bean sprouts, and most fruits and vegetables. Foods that have more arginine than lysine include gelatin, chocolate, carob, coconut, oats, whole wheat and white flour, peanuts, soybeans, and wheat germ. Best to stay away from those if you're having—or expecting—an outbreak. And if you want the therapeutic benefits of lysine for the prevention or control of herpes, it's best to take supplements. You're just not going to get nearly enough from food alone.

Everyday Prevention

Like many conditions discussed in this book, herpes has a very intimate relationship with stress. Stress makes it worse. A lot worse. Stress can actually bring on an outbreak, and it can certainly make an existing one worse.

Reducing stress is one of the best things you can do for yourself if you want to keep outbreaks to a minimum.

And while we're talking about prevention, keep in mind that using lysine as a preventive measure against cold sores without strengthening the overall immune system is a little like rearranging the deck chairs on the Titanic. The stronger your immune system, the less chance that the herpes virus will reemerge to wreak havoc on your social life. If the immune system is working properly, the herpes virus wouldn't find it quite so easy to get inside your cells, replicate, and ruin your chances to get a date Saturday night. Under normal conditions a healthy immune system would destroy the virus before it had a chance to do this. Vitamins like C and E are potent against the virus, and new research points to plant sterols as also playing a role by increasing natural killer cell activity (a good thing) and destroying the virus.

If you're prone to herpes of either variety, you should definitely give lysine a try. But don't stop there. The next time you get a cold sore—or even better, *before* you get one—think about reducing your stress level and increasing your immune-strengthening vitamins. And don't forget to sleep well. All of these factors will contribute to the prevention of a new herpes attack.

Natural Prescription for Herpes

Lysine: 1,000 to 3,000 mg (larger doses can be divided into 1,000 mg, three times per day)

Vitamin C and flavonoids: 200 mg of vitamin C plus 200 mg of flavonoids, each taken three to five times per day

Vitamin E: 400 IU, three times per day for three days and then cut back to 400 IU per day. Do not use if you are on anticoagulant drugs.

PLANT STEROLS:

Lemon balm (Melissa officinalis): Lemon balm cream applied two to four times per day for five to ten days

Topical tea tree oil ointment (not the undiluted oil) or

Licorice root gel: Applied to blisters as needed

Diet: Avoid foods that are high in arginine, such as nuts, peanuts, and chocolate. Eat foods high in lysine, such as Atlantic cod, beef, tofu, chicken, and turkey.

Note: All dosages are daily and in pill or capsule form unless otherwise noted.

Hot Flashes

Cool Down with Black Cohosh and Dong Quai

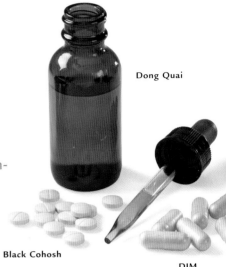

Dong Quai

Black Cohosh

DIM

OF ALL THE SYMPTOMS that accompany menopause, hot flashes would probably be at the top of the list of the most bothersome. Between 50 percent and 85 percent of U.S. women going through menopause experience hot flashes, and 40 percent of those women suffer from them severely enough to seek medical attention. Hot flashes, including night sweats, occur because of an imbalance in the ratios of two primary female hormones, estrogen and progesterone.

Black cohosh is a plant native to the United States and Canada and cultivated widely in Europe. That it has a medicinal effect is not in question; Native Americans used it for a wide variety of conditions, including menopausal symptoms. It's been used for pain and inflammation in Korean folk medicine. And the German Commission E has approved it for premenstrual discomfort. It's one of the best-selling herbs in the United States and a popular and accepted therapy in Europe.

A 2006 study in *Obstetrics and Gynecology* reported that a combination of St. John's Wort and black cohosh appears to be especially useful for women who suffer from menopause-related depression, especially interesting because recent research suggests that compounds in black cohosh bind to serotonin receptors in the brain. Another recent study in the journal *Gynecological Endocrinology* reported that black cohosh is as effective as the low-dose estrogen patch for relieving most symptoms and can also have a positive effect on cardiac risks.

"Since 2003 there have been about ten clinical studies on black cohosh, and all were positive," according to Gail Mahady, Ph.D., an associate professor of pharmacognosy at the University of Illinois and one of the principal authors of the black cohosh monograph for the World Health Organization.

One of the best-known commercial products containing a standardized extract of black cohosh is Remifemin, which seems to have an excellent track record in helping with hot flashes. The company's website (www.remifemin.com) explains what you can expect using a standardized black cohosh product and provides abstracts of research for those who want more information.

WORTH KNOWING

The position that menopause is a transition into a powerful and life-affirming stage of life is elucidated brilliantly, poetically, and movingly by my friend Christiane Northrup, M.D., in her excellent book *The Wisdom of Menopause*. Other wonderful books—notably the late Shari Lieberman's *Get Off the Menopause Roller Coaster!*—are also out there to help women navigate this transition in the healthiest and happiest of ways.

Natural Prescription for Hot Flashes

Black cohosh: The German product Remifemin uses an extract standardized to 1 mg of 27-deoxyactein per 20 mg tablet; *The British Herbal Compendium* recommends 40 to 200 mg dried rhizome daily in divided doses. Use each product as directed on package label.

Dong quai: Can be used together with black cohosh, as directed on product label

DIM (diindolylmethane): A balancer of estrogen metabolism, 100 to 200 mg per day

FOR ADDED EFFECTIVENESS:

Cruciferous vegetables: Cabbages, cauliflower, mustard greens, bok choy, broccoli, Brussels sprouts, radishes, and turnips

Flax/high fiber: Ground flaxseeds, any other fiber, 35 g

Fermented soy: Miso, tempeh, and natto

Vitamin E (mixed tocopherols or high-gamma tocopherol): 400 IU, twice daily. Up to 1,000 is fine, but do not increase if you are on anticoagulants.

Essential fatty acids: Evening primrose oil or gamma-linolenic acid (GLA) 250 to 500 mg

ALSO USEFUL:

Hormone therapy: Work with a health-care provider to determine appropriate levels. Choose natural hormones like Tri-Est, which contains all three forms of estrogens plus natural progesterone cream.

Acupuncture: Work with a qualified acupuncturist

Exercise: Studies show that hot flashes decrease immediately after aerobic exercise. Exercise also keeps you "happy" and increases bone density. Walking briskly every day for 30 minutes cuts hot flashes by 50 percent while improving your heart and bone health at the same time.

Note: The above dosages are daily and in pill or capsule form unless otherwise noted.

Other Plants Give Relief, Too

Dong quai has been used in Asian medicine for thousands of years and remains one of the most popular herbs in Chinese medicine where it is used primarily for "female" issues. It has even acquired a reputation as the "female ginseng." Despite its long tradition of use, the hard-core research on using dong quai for hot flashes—and other issues around menstruation and menopause—is weak.

It's worth noting, however, that in Chinese medicine, dong quai is almost always used in combination with other medicines and herbs. Dong quai may be one of those herbs or compounds that's used best as part of an overall treatment plan or formula, where it might have a synergistic effect. It doesn't seem to have too much of an effect on its own, though.

Soy has long had a reputation as being good for hot flashes. I wrote about soy in my book, *The 150 Healthiest Foods on Earth*, and if you read it, you probably know I'm not a big cheerleader for the "all soy all the time" brigade. (For one reason, the form in which we eat soy here in America—as soy junk food—bears little resemblance to the kind of soy in the traditional Asian diet.)

Fermented soy foods like miso and tempeh are fine. Asian women, who, by the way, have few menopausal symptoms, eat fermented soy as accompaniments to a nutrient-rich diet built around seafood and vegetables. If you walk around Tokyo, you won't find them consuming soy milk, soy yogurt, soy cheese, soy burgers, soy chicken, soy chips, and soy lasagna. Get my drift?

Bottom line: If you're going to eat soy, do as the Asians do. Don't overdo it and make sure it's fermented.

Hypertension/ High Blood Pressure

Get Your Levels Down with CoQ10, Whey Protein, and the DASH Diet

PRETTY MUCH EVERYTHING I know of value about hypertension I learned from Mark Houston, M.D., as did most of the nutritionists and doctors with whom I've trained. He's an associate clinical professor of medicine at Vanderbilt University School of Medicine and director of the Hypertension Institute in Nashville. In addition, he is a staff physician at Saint Thomas Medical Group and the Vascular Institute of Saint Thomas Hospital in Nashville. With both an M.D. and a master's degree in nutrition, he's uniquely qualified to speak about natural cures and the integration of conventional and nutritional medicine. And if you have hypertension, are at risk for it, or just want to know more, there's no better place to begin than with his book *What Your Doctor May Not Tell You about Hypertension.*

Green Pepper

Tomato

Beans

Lentils

CoQ10

Whey Protein Powder

The basics of Dr. Houston's Hypertension Institute Program involve a sophisticated vitamin regimen, exercise, weight maintenance, stress reduction, and the DASH diet (more on that in a moment). But several elements of the program stood out, and it's those three elements that form the core of our combo cure for hypertension: the DASH diet, coenzyme Q10, and hydrolyzed whey protein.

The DASH Diet

In 1997, the National Heart, Lung and Blood Institute funded research on the effects on blood pressure of groups of nutrients as they're found together in foods. The name of this study was Dietary Approaches to Stop Hypertension, or DASH, for short. The first study, known as DASH-1, investigated three dietary regimens: the standard American diet (with the apt acronym SAD), SAD plus some extra fruits and vegetables, and finally, the DASH-1 diet, which is high in fruits, vegetables, and low-fat dairy products, but low in cholesterol, saturated fat, and total fat. The results? Adding fruits and vegetables to the crummy SAD reduced blood pressure, demonstrating that simply eating more fruits and vegetables is helpful. But those on the DASH-1 diet enjoyed the greatest reduction in their blood pressure.

The thing of it was that the DASH-1 diet didn't control for sodium, and each of the three tested diets (including the DASH-1) contained about 3,000 mg of the stuff. So the researchers decided to do a second study, called the DASH-2 Sodium (or DASH-2 for short) diet. In this study, which involved both prehypertensives and hypertensives, half the subjects ate the DASH-2 diet; half ate the standard American diet (SAD). But every single subject consumed a specific level of sodium for one month at a time: 4,300 mg per day for the first month, 2,400 mg per day for the second month, and 1,500 mg per day for the third.

The results showed that simply cutting back on sodium intake reduced blood pressure, *no matter which diet a person followed*. But those on the DASH-2 diet showed *greater reductions* in blood pressure at each level of sodium restriction. And the *biggest* reductions were in those who were hypertensive when they started the diet.

Making Modifications

So we know that the DASH diet works for lowering blood pressure and works even better when you lower sodium in the diet as well. But at the Hypertension Institute, they've gone the DASH diet one better.

"I give my patients a specially modified version of the DASH that I believe is the best diet possible for people with hypertension," Houston told me. "The main change is to increase the amount of protein, vegetables, and 'good' fats consumed every day, while decreasing the grains, fruits, and dairy products. It's much lower in refined carbohydrates and has a lower glycemic index and glycemic load. Otherwise it's the same great, pressure-reducing program that's helped so many."

So here's what the best dietary "natural cure" for hypertension looks like:

- **Cereals, grains, pasta:** 3 to 4 servings a day, all from whole grains with no sugar or salt added
- **Vegetables:** 6 to 8 servings a day
- **Fruits:** 4 servings per day
- **Meat, poultry, and cold-water fish:** 2 to 4 servings per day

- **Dried beans, seeds, and nuts:** 1 to 2 servings per day
- **Low-fat dairy products:** 1 to 2 servings per day
- **Fats and oils:** 4 to 5 servings per day of polyunsaturated and monounsaturated fats; no trans fats; low saturated fat
- **Sweets:** none
- **Fiber:** mixed (soluble and insoluble) 50 g a day

(You can read more about the specifics of this diet in Houston's book, mentioned above.)

Note: With all this talk about salt and the dangers of sodium for people with high blood pressure, it's important to note that this is not true for everyone. Houston estimates that up to 60 percent of those with elevated blood pressure are salt sensitive—that is, their blood pressure rises when they consume more salt and falls when they take in less. African Americans, the elderly, and the obese are more likely to be salt sensitive. But many people are not.

Couple the DASH diet, especially in its Houston-modified form (above), with a couple of superstar nutrients, add exercise and some form of stress reduction and you're well on your way to making a big difference in your health.

Here are the superstar nutrients that form the basis of the combo cure for hypertension.

CoEnzyme Q10. Coenzyme Q10 is widely given in Europe and Japan to millions of people suffering from cardiovascular disease. People with essential hypertension are more likely to have a CoQ10 deficiency than those without hypertension. It's been an approved treatment for congestive heart failure in Japan since 1974, and Houston considers it one of the best natural treatments for high blood pressure.

Whey Protein Powder. In addition to being a superb source of high-quality, absorbable protein, hydrolyzed whey protein is a natural ACE inhibitor. ACE inhibitors, short for angiotensin-converting enzyme inhibitors, help reduce blood pressure by interfering with an enzyme that causes muscles surrounding the arteries to constrict, thus raising blood pressure. "Hydrolyzed whey protein lowers blood pressure," says Houston.

The Supporting Cast

Though CoQ10, whey protein, and the DASH diet form the core of a natural cure for high blood pressure, they're far from the only elements of a hypertension reduction program. Calcium, magnesium, and potassium (and a reduced amount of sodium) work in concert to optimize blood pressure. Much research has shown that the overwhelming majority of Americans are deficient in magnesium, so supplementing with magnesium makes a great deal of sense. And as far back as 1928, studies have suggested that a high potassium intake could reduce elevated blood pressure. Since then, numerous population, observational, and clinical studies have demonstrated that blood pressure falls when dietary potassium is increased.

Omega-3 fatty acids are the kind of fats that can help lower blood pressure the most and improve overall heart health to boot. And especially in people with high blood pressure, vitamin C improves endothelial dysfunction (a dysfunction of the cells that line the inner surface of all blood vessels) in people with hypertension.

Natural Prescription for Hypertension

DASH diet: Houston modification

Coenzyme Q10: 50 to 300 mg

Hydrolyzed whey protein powder: 1 serving of 30 g

FOR ADDED EFFECTIVENESS:

Magnesium chelate: 500 mg, twice a day

Calcium citrate: 1,000 mg

Taurine: 1,500 mg, twice a day

Omega-3 fatty acids: 2 to 3 g

Vitamin D: 2,000 IU

L-arginine: 2 g twice a day

L-carnitine: 1,500 to 4,000 mg per day in divided doses

High-quality multiple vitamin with vitamin E and vitamin C

ALSO RECOMMENDED:

Exercise

Stress reduction

Celery, garlic, and extra virgin olive oil

Hawthorne berries: 80 to 300 mg per day

Note: All dosages are daily dosages and in pill or capsule form unless otherwise noted.

A diet high in fruits and vegetables can do wonders for high blood pressure, possibly because they are so high in magnesium and potassium. Certain foods are especially helpful. Celery, for example, can lower blood pressure when you consume four sticks a day. So can garlic.

Finally, resveratrol has made news for the last decade or so as one of the key "antiaging" compounds in red wine and grapes. "It lowers blood pressure, blood fats, and glucose," Houston says, "and it relaxes the vascular smooth muscles." And just in case you were living on another planet for the last few decades—stop smoking. Immediately. Do it now. No excuses.

(For more information about the full hypertension reduction program of supplements and lifestyle changes, visit www.hypertensioninstitute.com.)

Impotence/Erectile Dysfunction/ Sagging Libido

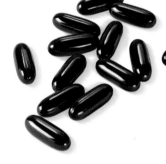

Get Your Old Self Back with Horny Goat Weed

LET'S BE CLEAR. Impotence has multiple causes. If you're not turned on by your partner, if you're depressed, or if you've got a ton of things on your mind, you may not be in the mood for love. It's unlikely that any supplement on the planet is going to make you suddenly fall in lust with Miss Anderson in accounting, particularly if you can't stand her to begin with. But if circulation or blood flow is an issue, there are some natural cures that may indeed give your sex life a boost.

Ever hear of Epimedium sagittatum? Me, either. But this herb, found throughout Asia and the Mediterranean, goes by another name in the United States, one you might recognize if you've thumbed through the ads in men's magazines in the last few years: horny goat weed.

Legend has it that this plant got its nickname from a goat herder who happened to notice that his flock would graze on this herb and then get noticeably more, well, frisky. Also known as yin yang huo, epimedium has a long history in Chinese medicine as a tonic for the liver, joints, and kidneys. But in the United States, its principal use is as an aphrodisiac.

What Do the Chinese Know That We Don't?

Horny goat weed is loaded with flavonoids, polysaccharides, sterols, and an alkaloid called magnaflorine, according to herbal medicine expert Chris Kilham, author of the *Hot Plants: Nature's Proven Sex Boosters for Men and Women*. This time-tested aphrodisiac "increases libido in men and women, and improves erectile function in men," Kilham says.

Kilham went to China to interview traditional Chinese medicine practitioners for the Discovery Channel, and was told by Diao Yuan Kuang, M.D., that horny goat weed "… gives you back your sexual strength." Chinese doctors use it to treat erectile problems, boost libido, and recapture the sexual vitality of youth. Herb traders in China estimate that they sell more than 100 tons of the stuff every year.

Little research has been done on horny goat weed and libido, but it has a long history of successful use, and many health practitioners, not only in Asia, but over here, endorse it. "Epimedium is, in fact, likely to make you horny. Most users will notice a mild to moderate effect on the third or fourth day of use," says Ray Sahelian, M.D., author of *Natural Sex Boosters*.

Kilham, who's my go-to guy for exotic herbal products, recommends supplements that are standardized to a flavonoid called *icarlin*. Two to four 500 mg capsules per day should be enough to help with libido and heat up your sex life.

Peruvian Ginseng

Maca, also known as "Peruvian ginseng," has been used for sex enhancement since the time of the Incas. It's actually a radish-shaped vegetable that grows well in the Andes Mountains. I first heard about maca when I interviewed a researcher on my New York radio show who found that feeding maca to rodents increased their spontaneous erections. (This study was published in the April 2000 issue of the medical journal *Urology*.) Maca root contains a chemical called p-methoxybenzyl isothiocyanate, which is reputed to have aphrodisiac qualities. (It also contains a bunch of chemicals found in other plants from the Brassica family (broccoli, cabbage, etc.), which are document-ed to be cancer preventive.)

Other research has demonstrated increased sexual activity in mice that are fed maca, though some of this research has been criticized because it was performed and sponsored by people marketing maca. But there's been some human research as well, notably by G.F. Gonzales et al., published in the *Asian Journal of Andrology*. Men aged twenty-one to fifty-six received either a placebo, 1,500 mg of maca, or 3,000 mg of maca. Sperm count and semen volume were increased with maca at either dose.

Why the effects? Who knows? Maca contains two novel groups of compounds—*macamides* and *macaenes*, which may be responsible for its effects. Maca also contains the amino acid L-arginine (see below), which has been shown to increase sperm production and motility and is necessary for the creation of nitric oxide, a molecule that is necessary for erections. (More on nitric oxide in a moment.)

"For the Sex, of Course!"

An interesting theory on maca and sexual activity has to do with the fact that maca contains high amounts of an amino acid called histidine. Histidine plays an often-overlooked role in both ejaculation and orgasm. It gets tricky here, but stay with me. The body uses histidine to produce histamine. High levels of histamine are often found in men who have premature ejaculation. (That's one reason why a side effect of antihistamines is difficulty in achieving orgasm.) According to the Tropical Plant Database website, a prohistamine like maca might have exactly the opposite effect of an antihistamine. It might make it easier for men and women who have trouble reaching orgasm to achieve it.

Regardless of the science, the proof is in the pudding. Kilham, investigating maca in Peru on one of his frequent "Medicine Hunter" expeditions, asked a number of people why they used maca. "One woman stands out in my mind," he says. "She smiled at my question and replied, 'Well, for the sex, of course.'"

Then there's L-arginine. Though no cure for impotence, L-arginine has a documented role in the body as a vasodilator, benefiting circulation and helping with endothelial dysfunction, a dysfunction of cells that line the inner surface of blood vessels. (Endothelial dysfunction is often a predictor of later vascular events like heart attacks and strokes.) What's the connection to sexual performance? Simple: circulation.

"I've almost never seen a case of erectile dysfunction that didn't also have a component of the other ED—endothelial dysfunction," says Mark Houston, M.D. "They frequently go together."

The claim for arginine as a natural treatment for erectile dysfunction is that it increases levels of another molecule in the body, the previous mentioned nitric oxide.

"No" Means "Yes" for Your Heart and Your Libido

Nitric oxide (abbreviation NO) was named "molecule of the year" by *Science* magazine in 1992. Its discovery led to the Nobel Prize in 1998 and has led to an explosion of research about it ever since. Briefly, this signaling molecule tells the arteries to "relax and expand," which is why it's so vital for healthy circulation. Viagra actually works because it improves nitric oxide signaling in the penis. (And no, I'm not making that up.)

The claim for arginine is that it increases NO in the body, but according to Nathan Bryan, Ph.D., of the School of Medicine of University of Texas Health Science Center (and co-author of *The Nitrous Oxide Solution*), we don't break down arginine very well after the age of 40. Bryan suggests a better solution to increasing NO stores, which is a supplement called NEO 40 (available at www.neogenis.com).

Nitric oxide won't turn you into a young Johnny Depp, but if circulation issues are stalling your libido, it might be the thing to get your engine going.

Natural Prescription for Impotence/Erectile Dysfunction/Sagging Libido

Horny goat weed, standardized to 10 percent icarlin: 2 to 4 500 mg capsules

Maca: 1,800 to 2,500 mg

L-arginine: 1,000 to 2,000 mg (or NEO40, 1 lozenge daily under the tongue)

Zinc: 25 mg

Note: All dosages are daily dosages and come in pill or capsule form unless otherwise noted.

Infection Prevention

Stay Healthy with Zinc

IF MINERALS WERE ancient gods, zinc would be Zeus: superhero mineral, protector of the immune system, defender of bodily invaders, and involved in virtually every aspect of infection prevention. If you've got a cold or an infection, zinc may just be your best friend.

Critical for more than 300 enzymatic functions in the body, zinc is found in every one of our 80 trillion cells. Without it we wouldn't survive. Zinc helps us grow and develop, breathe, and digest our food. One of its primary functions is in wound healing and tissue repair. In the language of the twenty-first century, it is a "healing" nutrient. Because our bodies are constantly being subjected to little injuries (and big ones), we need zinc for the rebuilding process (healing). Without it, we'd simply break down.

If you're like millions of people in America, you're likely to reach for zinc lozenges at the first sign of a cold. That would be smart. A study at the famous Cleveland Clinic showed that zinc lozenges decreased the duration of colds by an impressive 50 percent.

The Natural Standard database, one of the most respected sources of supplement and medical data I know of, rates the evidence of a positive effect for zinc on the immune system a very respectable B, meaning "strong scientific evidence." Considering that getting a B from the Natural Standard is like getting a B at Harvard, I'd say that's pretty good.

Zinc possesses antiviral activity and will attack viruses that may cause the common cold. The *American Journal of Clinical Nutrition* reported a recent study demonstrating that after one year of either zinc supplementation or no supplementation, those taking zinc experienced far fewer colds than those who took a placebo. In addition, 88 percent of participants in a study of the elderly developed colds when they didn't take 45 mg of zinc regularly. Note that these participants ranged in age from 55 to 87—it's very possible that we need higher levels of zinc as we age.

Zinc lozenges became popular after a well-publicized 2000 study done at Wayne State University in Detroit showed that they significantly reduced the duration of the common cold. They work because they bathe the throat tissues where viruses multiply. So reach for zinc lozenges during cold and flu season.

Nixing the Naysayers

Of course, like most natural treatments, zinc has its naysayers. One study in particular is widely touted by the anti-supplement brigade as evidence that zinc has no effect on the common cold. But let's go to the videotape. Three dosages of zinc were given to subjects with colds—5 mg, 11.5 mg, and 13.3 mg. These amounts are pretty paltry; 5 mg isn't even 65 percent of the recommended daily allowance (RDA) for women, and it's less than *half* of what's recommended for healthy men. (It could reasonably be assumed that sick folks might need *more* than the RDA.) When the researchers "averaged" the results for all three groups, sure enough these little bitty doses of zinc didn't make a difference.

However, for the group getting the 13.3 mg dose, the duration of the cold was about 30 percent shorter. I don't know about you, but if a tiny drop of zinc cuts my cold length by a day—which happened in this study—I'm taking it.

This study also used two different types of zinc—zinc acetate and zinc gluconate, and only one was effective (the gluconate). The lesson here isn't that zinc has no effect on the common cold, it's that you've got to use the right amount and the right type of zinc. Note: To alleviate cold symptoms, for several days try lozenges providing 13 to 23 mg of zinc gluconate or zinc gluconate-glycine every two hours while awake. The best effect is obtained when lozenges are used at the first sign of a cold.

Zinc: The Missing Link for Superimmunity

Studies have shown that severe zinc deficiency significantly depresses immune function because zinc is needed for both the development and the activation of a very important class of white blood cells (lymphocytes) called T cells. When people with low zinc are given zinc supplements, their T-cell count goes up and they're better able to fight off disease.

There's a fair amount of research showing that malnourished children given zinc supplements have shorter courses of infectious diarrhea. Zinc supplements also can help heal skin ulcers and bedsores for people who are low in zinc to begin with. (When zinc levels are normal, however, supplements don't seem to make the wounds heal any faster.)

Problem is, how do you know when your levels are normal? You don't. There's no single laboratory test that consistently and accurately measures zinc status. Nutritionists, however, have used a test for years called the *zinc taste test*. Here's how to do it at home: First you get some liquid zinc. (Liquid zinc is available at better health food stores or through health practitioners. You can't use a flavored kind—it has to be pure, clear, and tasteless, like Zinc Talley by Metagenics.) The test is simple: You just hold a capful or two of the liquid zinc in your mouth for about a minute. If it tastes like metal, you're not zinc deficient. But if it tastes like water, you are.

One thing we know for sure is this: Most of us don't get nearly enough zinc. According to the U.S. Department of Agriculture's 1996 Continuing Survey of Food Intakes, more than 70 percent of Americans don't consume the recommended daily allowance, which is only 8 mg a day for women and 11 mg a day for men. (Ten percent of individuals don't even consume half the RDA!)

Emily Ho, Ph.D., a research scientist at Linus Pauling Institute of Oregon State University, estimates that zinc deficiency affects more than 2 billion people worldwide, about one-third of the entire planet. Liping Huang, a geneticist at the ARS Western Human Nutrition Research Center at Davis, California, notes that "mild zinc deficiency may exist in the United States among otherwise healthy infants, toddlers, preschool children, pregnant and lactating women, and seniors." People who avoid meat and dairy are also at risk for mild zinc deficiencies.

A Little Goes a Long Way

And zinc isn't one of those nutrients you need to "oversupplement" with. You can do really well with supplementing in the 15 to 50 mg range, although for some situations (like macular degeneration or fighting off a cold or healing a wound) it's perfectly okay to use a higher dose for a short time. In general, a basic 15 mg a day seems to help fend off most common problems. Certain seafoods, notably oysters, along with milk, whole grain breads, dark meat poultry, and nuts like cashews also provide plenty of the mineral.

A number of factors can interfere with zinc absorption, such as chemical compounds called phytates that are found in cereals and soy foods and bind to minerals like zinc, keeping them from being absorbed. Even fiber may decrease zinc's availability. Stress definitely depletes it, and very easily!

Another Weapon in the Immunity Arsenal: Olive Leaf Complex

Olive leaf complex is another supplement worthy of consideration if you're trying to keep your immune system in tip top shape. That's because olives are loaded with plant compounds called *polyphenols*. Polyphenols are a group of valuable chemicals found throughout the plant kingdom primarily in berries, walnuts, olives, tea, grapes, and other fruits and vegetables. These polyphenols also have antimicrobial activity against a wide variety of viruses, bacteria, yeasts, and fungi.

Scientific advances have shown that there are at least 30 distinct polyphenols in fresh-picked olive leafs and that the *full spectrum of these polyphenols* in fresh-picked olive leaves gives a synergistic effect greater than any individual isolated compound alone. This is why the most bio-effective olive leaf products (such as Barlean's Olive Leaf Complex) are always made directly from fresh-picked, whole olive leaves which provide the *whole spectrum* of natural polyphenolic antioxidants just as nature intended. This also enables them to work together in natural synergy to maximize the health benefits.

The bitter substances in olive leaves, the polyphenols *oleuropein*, *hydroxytyrosol*, *caffeic acid*, *verbascoside*, etc., have been found to be particularly helpful in resisting bacterial damage. In fact, early research by the drug company Upjohn found extracts from olive leaves to be effective in treating infection by a large number of viruses as well as bacteria and parasitic protozoans.

In vitro studies have found that olive leaf extract is effective against more than fifty common disease-causing organisms, including herpes, influenza A, Polio 1, 2, and 3; *Salmonella typhimurium*, *Candida Krusei* and *Cox-sackie* A 21.

Biochemist Arnold Takemoto, talking to the *Townsend Newsletter for Doctors and Patients*, put it this way: "(I have) yet to discover another herbal substance that accomplishes antimicrobially what this substance achieves."

What Dosage is Best?

Though there is really no "official" recommended dose for taking olive leaf complex, many experts recommend a basic maintenance dose for general use and a "therapeutic" dose for special cases. Generally, the consensus is that one tablespoonful (15ml) one to two times a day taken right before eating is ideal for maintenance.

For conditions such as the common cold, flu, sinus infections, and basic respiratory tract infections, the recommended dose is two 5 ml teaspoons every six hours," says naturopath Jack Ritchason, N.D. For acute infections such as sore throat, swollen glands, or fever, Ritchason recommends three teaspoons (15 ml) every six hours.

On a personal note, I take a capful of Barlean's Olive Leaf Complex on a daily basis as a general tonic and immune system booster. Although this is hardly a scientific statement, I can tell you that I rarely get sick and on the few occasions that I do, it's very mild and I'm back to my routine in record time. Apparently, I'm not alone in being a fan of olive leaf complex. Experts agree that taking this wonderful supplement can be a valuable part of anyone's health routine.

Says Ritchason, "From all indications—research, case studies, and widespread use—olive leaf extract appears to be an extremely safe supplement that can effectively aid the body in improving immune function and fighting infection by various microbes."

Amen to that.

Infertility
Try One of the Oldest Treatments on Earth

HAVING TROUBLE GETTING PREGNANT? You might want to consider acupuncture. Acupuncture might not be the first thing you think of if you're having a problem with infertility, but maybe it should be. Studies—and a great deal of clinical experience—suggest that it might help, even if you're already undergoing standard therapies like in vitro fertilization or intrauterine insemination.

Acupuncture is actually one of the oldest medical practices in the world. Although it originated in China more than two millennia ago, it first gained popularity in the United States when a well-known and respected *New York Times* reporter named James Reston wrote glowingly about it after it helped ease his postsurgical pain. As of this writing, more than 8 million American adults have had acupuncture treatment. As practiced by licensed practitioners who undergo extensive training and are often trained in traditional Chinese medicine (TCM) as well, it is completely safe and quite effective for a number of conditions. One of those conditions is infertility.

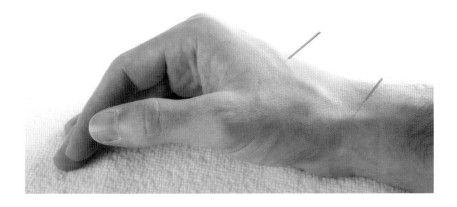

The Yin, the Yang, and Baby Makes Three

Acupuncture, like TCM, is based on a concept of the body as a balance of forces—yin (the cold, the slow, and the passive) and yang (the hot, the excited, and the active). The general theory of acupuncture is based on the premise that vital energy (known as qi or chi) flows along pathways in the body, that there are patterns of this energy flow that are essential for health, and that disruptions of this flow are responsible for disease. Optimal health is achieved when energy is in balance, flowing effortlessly through the body. Qi travels through twenty major pathways, which TCM calls "meridians." They're accessible through 400 different acupuncture points. By stimulating these meridians at carefully chosen points and in carefully chosen combinations, the acupuncturist can overcome blocks, help balance energy, and promote health.

One of the reasons conventional Western medicine has trouble wrapping its mind around acupuncture is that it's hard to subject it to the kind of specific scientific study that Western scientists are used to. In a standard scientific study, one group is given a drug (the experimental group) and the other group (the placebo group) is given a sugar pill. No one knows who gets what, including the researchers measuring the results (hence the description "double blind"). The researchers then observe whether there's a difference in some variable of interest (cholesterol, blood pressure, and so on), and whether the difference is great enough, they attribute it to the pill. But how do you give the "sugar pill" equivalent of acupuncture? You can put the needles in neutral places (called a "sham" treatment) and compare it to the "real" treatment, but this isn't a perfect solution and there's a lot of disagreement about how to do it.

In addition, Western medicine doesn't really have a concept that's equivalent to "energy." For left-brained Western doctors, you either see something or you don't. If it's not measurable and observable, they're usually not interested. Acupuncture—for many conservative, rigid thinkers trained conventionally in Western medicine—is just plain weird. But that's changing. In 1997, a blue ribbon panel at the National Institutes of Health issued a statement on acupuncture that said, in part: "[P]romising results have emerged, for example, showing efficacy of acupuncture in adult postoperative and chemotherapy nausea and vomiting and in postoperative dental pain. There are other situations such as addiction, stroke rehabilitation, headache, menstrual cramps, tennis elbow, fibromyalgia, myofascial pain, osteoarthritis, low back pain, carpal tunnel syndrome, and asthma, in which acupuncture may be useful as an adjunct treatment or an acceptable alternative or be included in a comprehensive management program. Further research is likely to uncover additional areas where acupuncture interventions will be useful."

Indeed, one of those areas of "further research" has been infertility. And the results have been hard to argue with.

The Causes of Infertility

Two basic types of problems can interfere with fertility: structural problems (e.g., damaged fallopian tubes) or functional problems (e.g., an irregular menstrual cycle).

"By needling certain points on the meridians you can influence and rebalance the endocrine and hormonal system," says Cindy Lawrence, LAc, a licensed acupuncturist who also holds a master's degree in Oriental medicine. "Regulating the menstrual cycle is very important—maybe the patient is not ovulating or [her] luteal phase is too short." Lawrence points out that together with the traditional Chinese herbs often used by acupuncturists as complements to the treatment, acupuncture can increase blood flow to the uterus, further increasing the chances of successful implantation.

Then, of course, there's the stress connection.

A running theme throughout this book is the effect stress can have on many health conditions. Stress hormones wreak havoc with virtually every metabolic process, influencing everything from weight to brain function. And acupuncture really shines when it comes to reducing stress.

"If energy is stagnated or out of balance in certain meridians or organs it can result in stress and anxiety," Lawrence explains. Patients typically report an almost otherworldly, completely pleasant feeling of relaxation after a session. (For what it's worth, that's been my experience the dozen or so times I've tried acupuncture. You literally can fall asleep on the table, and invariably sleep like a baby afterward.)

Then there's the research, and it's pretty impressive. One study in Germany compared a group of eighty women undergoing in vitro fertilization with eighty women undergoing the same treatment plus acupuncture. Only twenty-one of the women who received only in vitro fertilization became pregnant (26.3 percent), but thirty-four of the women who also received acupuncture conceived (42.5 percent). An American study produced equally impressive results. Fifty-one percent of those who had the additional acupuncture treatment became pregnant, while only 36 percent of those receiving only in vitro fertilization did. In addition, fewer than half as many who received acupuncture miscarried.

Yet another study, done at Women's Hospital at the University of Heidelberg, Germany, involved forty-five infertile women. Following a complete gynecological and endocrinologic exam, they were treated with acupuncture. Their results compared with those of a matched sample of forty-five women of the same age and history who had been treated with conventional hormones. The women treated with hormones had twenty pregnancies (and a number of side effects). The women treated with acupuncture? Twenty-two pregnancies (and no side effects).

Finally, a study at the Fertility Clinic Trianglen in Denmark concluded that "acupuncture … significantly improves the reproductive outcome of IVF (in vitro fertilization) and ICSI (intracytoplasmic sperm injection) compared to no acupuncture."

Best of all, acupuncture for infertility is truly a "whole person" treatment that looks at the woman as much more than just a dysfunctional reproductive system. "People come into my office and they're completely unprepared for conception," Lawrence told me. "They're overworked, sleep deprived, not happy, overweight, and stressed out, which is not the best environment for a conception or a pregnancy."

Lawrence spends considerable time with the women who come to see her, making sure they take time to relax, eat the right foods, and manage their stress and sleep. She prescribes herbs on a completely individual basis to strengthen the areas of the patient's body that are not in balance. "It's very important in Chinese medicine to prepare the body—you don't plant a seed in infertile ground," she says.

Oh, one more thing in case you're wondering—acupuncture doesn't hurt a bit. If you closed your eyes during the treatment, you'd never even know that there were needles actually sticking out of you. I know this for a fact because I've had it done. Obviously it didn't make me pregnant—but it definitely felt good afterward.

Inflammatory Bowel Disease (Crohn's Disease/ Ulcerative Colitis)

Ease Your Symptoms with the Specific Carbohydrate Diet and These Supplements

INFLAMMATORY BOWEL DISEASE (IBD) is the collective name for two diseases in which the intestines become deeply inflamed: Crohn's disease and ulcerative colitis. Unlike irritable bowel syndrome, in both forms of inflammatory bowel disease there is active pathology in the tissues.

If you have IBD, a biopsy of your tissue would come back with visible, active inflammation, which would not be the case in irritable bowel syndrome.

Though there are similarities between Crohn's and ulcerative colitis, there are also differences, mainly in the location of the inflammation. Crohn's can affect you anywhere, from the mouth through the anus, and usually causes sores along the length of the small and large intestines. Ulcerative colitis always begins in the rectum, extends for a bit, and then stops. There's a clear "line of demarcation" between the tissue that is affected and the tissue that's not. It's characteristic of ulcerative colitis that usually just the mucosa and submucosa are involved, whereas in Crohn's all layers of the bowel are involved. Crohn's has "skip spaces"—that is, unaffected areas interspersed between involved areas. Ulcerative colitis does not; it's one contiguous inflammation for however long it extends from the rectum (it is confined to the rectum in about 25 percent of cases). Crohn's usually "spares" the rectum, but not always.

According to William Shapiro, M.D., of the Scripps Clinic and Research Foundation, about 20 percent of patients have a clinical picture that falls somewhere between ulcerative colitis and Crohn's—they are said to have "indeterminate colitis." As of this writing, about 1 million people are thought to have IBD in the United States. Both can cause extreme bouts of watery (Crohn's) or bloody (ulcerative colitis) diarrhea and abdominal pain.

The exact cause of IBD is not known, but like most multifaceted, highly complex disorders, it probably has a genetic component and is certainly made worse by trigger foods, bad nutrition in general, and stress. It's more common among whites, and it's higher in Ashkenazi Jews than in other groups, and slightly higher rates are seen in females. Antibiotic exposure has been mentioned as a possible factor, as have food sensitivities (more on that in a moment).

It's unlikely that any one factor "causes" IBD, but it's very likely that there's an interaction among factors. That said, it makes sense to support the immune system and remove as many potential triggers from the diet as possible. It also makes sense to reduce stress and to manage any secondary symptoms like depression.

The Specific Carbohydrate Diet

Thousands of people have used with success the Specific Carbohydrate Diet, or SCD. Developed by Elaine Gottschall, it's based on the theory that a balance in intestinal flora (good and bad bacteria) is absolutely essential to the health of the digestive system, and that an overgrowth of the "bad" bacteria like yeast leads to an imbalance in the gut that can create havoc. These "bad" bacteria create their own waste products and toxins and interfere with digestion and absorption of carbohydrates, which in turn leaves undigested carbohydrates to remain in the gut and become food for the microbes we host. The microbes digest these unused carbohydrates through the process of fermentation, creating waste products and acids that irritate and damage the gut.

Gottschall believed that some individuals with intestinal disease can't digest certain carbohydrates known as disaccharides (a kind of sugar). She believed that some individuals have impaired ability to break down disaccharides and that certain bacteria and yeast thrive on these molecules, creating a "vicious cycle" that can only be broken by changing the diet. The SCD is based on the principle that "specifically selected carbohydrates requiring minimal digestive processes, are well absorbed and leave virtually none to be used for furthering microbial overgrowth in the intestine," she wrote.

The guidelines for the Specific Carbohydate Diet are, well, very specific. And they have to be followed for a year before adding in any other foods. But thousands of people swear by the diet's effectiveness. General guidelines are no grains (e.g., rice, wheat, corn, or oats); no processed foods; no starchy vegetables (e.g., potatoes and yams); no canned vegetables of any kind; no flour, sugar, or sweeteners other than honey and saccharin; and no milk products except for homemade yogurt fermented for 24 hours.

Other Dietary Interventions

The Specific Carbohydrate Diet is a specialized version of a more generalized approach that has been used with some success for a number of digestive and gastrointestinal problems. Joe Brasco, M.D., a gastroenterologist with a decidedly holistic and nutritional bent, puts all his patients on a foundational program that is a basic "caveman"-type diet: lean meats, fish, poultry, vegetables and vegetable juices, stocks, and traditionally fermented foods like sauerkraut. He also recommends coconut oil because of its high content of lauric acid, a natural antimicrobial. The only dairy products he recommends are the highest-quality cultured dairy products from sheep or goats (yogurt).

"I wish I could tell you that I see people get completely off medications 100 percent of the time using this kind of dietary approach," Brasco says, "but I see it at least 10 percent of the time. And that tells me there's a significant subset of the population who responds unbelievably well to this intervention." Brasco uses the rule of thirds: "Using diet, lifestyle, and supplements, about one-third of patients will get off all medications. About one-third will be able to reduce their medications. And about one-third won't be helped. But a dietary plan like this doesn't cost anything. What's the downside of trying it?"

Alan Gaby, M.D., one of the leaders of the complementary medicine movement in America, is even more bullish about the success rate when treating patients with dietary modification and nutritional supplementation. "In my experience," he says, "at least half of the patients with Crohn's disease improve, and many become completely symptom-free."

A high-fiber diet is highly recommended for both types of inflammatory bowel disease, *except* when there is an active flare-up (during which you might have to go easy and actually eat *less* fiber till the flare-up subsides). The problem is that a lot of people associate high fiber with wheat, grains, and cereals, which may be exactly what you *don't* need (see below). A good idea would be to increase fiber as much as possible from vegetables, seeds, nuts, and even fiber supplements like psyllium husks. (You might want to lightly steam or cook the vegetables if eating them raw is a problem.) Drink plenty of water— a good idea in any event, but especially important when you're increasing fiber in your diet.

"Dietary fiber has a profound effect on the intestinal environment," says Michael Murray, N.D., a noted naturopath and the author of *The Encyclopedia of Natural Medicine*.

If you suffer with Crohn's or Ulcerative Colitis and find the Specific Carbohydrate Diet too daunting, a good first step would be to eliminate dairy (cow's milk protein), as well as wheat and other gluten-containing grains (barley, rye). These are two of the top triggers for food intolerance and sensitivities, and removing them may give some symptom relief.

Three Essential Supplements: Probiotics, Vitamin D, and Fish Oil

Regardless of whether you buy the exact theory behind Gottschall's SCD, the balance in intestinal flora between "good" and "bad" bacteria is essential for good health and especially for good digestion and absorption of nutrients. A high-quality probiotic formula is absolutely essential. Several research studies have shown significant improvement in people with inflammatory bowel disease who were put on probiotics.

Vitamin D deficiency is common in people suffering from intestinal malabsorption. The Cedars-Sinai website gives vitamin D supplements a three-star rating (its highest) for Crohn's disease, meaning there is reliable and consistent scientific data showing a health benefit. Nearly every practitioner I spoke to about natural treatments for IBD mentioned vitamin D supplements as essential.

Finally, fish oil, which contains two important omega-3 fatty acids that are highly anti-inflammatory, is also a must. No matter what else is going on, inflammatory bowel disease always has a huge inflammation component, so natural anti-inflammatories like fish oil are important to take on a daily basis. If you are allergic to fish, by all means use flaxseed oil—at least a tablespoon per 100 pounds of body weight.

Natural Prescription for Inflammatory Bowel Disease

SPECIFIC CARBOHYDRATE DIET

Essential fatty acids: 2 to 4 g

Probiotics: 10 to 20 billion

Vitamin D: 2,000 IU (or more if advised by health professional)

MAY ALSO BE HELPFUL:

L-glutamine: 3 to 6 g

Digestive enzymes: Taken as directed with each meal

Boswellia (optional): 1,200 mg, three times a day (extract standardized to 37.5 percent boswellic acids per dose)

Aloe vera: 800 to 1,600 mg (look for a product with high content of acemannan)

Note: All dosages are daily dosages and in pill or capsule form unless otherwise noted.

Insomnia/Sleep Disorders

Rest Easy with Inositol

LOOK UP "SLEEP DISORDER" on Wikipedia and you'll get no fewer than seventeen different entries ranging from *bruxism* (grinding your teeth) to *snoring*. (There's even one called *sexsomnia*. Give up? It means "sleep sex." And no, I did not make that up.) All of the disorders have one thing in common: They interfere with a good night's sleep. And that can spell serious problems indeed.

Many important things happen during sleep. Your brain makes certain hormones (melatonin and human growth hormone, for example) and replenishes vital biochemicals that keep you performing at your best during the day. Lack of sleep has been implicated in everything from obesity to traffic accidents. (It's well known that the day of the year with the greatest number of traffic accidents is the day after Daylight Saving Time ends.)

Sleep disorders are big business. As of this writing, use of sleep medications has grown by more than 60 percent since 2000, and in 2006, makers of sleeping pills spent more than $600 million advertising directly to consumers. Obviously, more than a few people are having some problems catching some good shut-eye.

Inositol might be the answer. This interesting substance is usually considered a member of the B vitamin family, but it's not technically a vitamin (it contains no nitrogen) and it's synthesized by the human body. No matter. This terrific little compound has multiple uses, one of which is that it's absolutely terrific for inducing sleep. What's more, it has none of the side effects of sleep medications. You're not likely to wake up in your kitchen in the middle of an ice cream raid. And you're also not likely to feel drowsy and bleary in the morning.

Inositol is "nature's sleeping pill." Taken before bedtime, it can significantly improve sleep quality. People who take it report a general relaxed feeling akin to having a few calming "sleepy-time" teas.

On "Insomnia Forum," one anonymous Internet poster reported this after adding 1,500 to 2,000 mg of inositol to his bedtime routine: "I'm not sure if it's the inositol, but this is the best sleep I've had in over two years of severe insomnia. It's the refreshing kind too, not the shallow type I've gotten on sleeping pills or other drugs." Normally I wouldn't repeat an anonymous Internet posting, but I've heard this sort of thing from many people over the years and I've experienced it myself.

Though we don't know exactly why inositol works so well as a sleeping aid, most researchers who are aware of its effects assume it's because inositol is involved in the serotonin pathways. Serotonin, the "relaxing" neurotransmitter, is out of balance in many mental health disturbances, such as depression, panic disorder, and obsessive-compulsive disorder (OCD). Interesting, then, that inositol has been used—albeit in small studies—with good results in treating all three of these disorders. One study in 1996 showed a significant improvement in OCD patients when they were given 18 g of inositol a day. And in a double-blind, controlled crossover test, 12 g of inositol was shown to be as effective in treating panic disorder as the medication Luvox, though without the typical side effects of nausea and tiredness.

Inositol is completely safe. Though you can take it in capsule form (1,500 to 2,000 mg seems to be good for sleep induction), I recommend (and prefer) the powdered form because it mixes easily in water, tastes pretty bland, and makes it way easier to get a significant dose (like 6 or 7 g). Just to get used to it, start with about 1/4 to 1/2 teaspoon (roughly 3/4 of a gram to 11/2 g) and work up to the dose that makes you feel best and gives you the best night's sleep. A few teaspoons should do it easily. (It's been used safely up to 18 g and is probably safe in amounts even greater than that, though you won't need that much.)

Natural Prescription for Insomnia

Drink 2 g of powdered inositol in water before bedtime. Alternately (or in addition) take one pack iSleep HerbPac.

Chinese Herbs Can Help

I'll be honest—I've had my own share of trouble sleeping and am always on the lookout for natural formulas that might help. While attending the annual Conference on Evidence-Based Supplements at the Scripps Center in southern California one year, I was introduced to a product I'd never seen before: a formulation of Chinese herbs sold by a wonderful small company called PAC herbs.

I tried it. It worked. And I love it.

Asian countries commonly treat insomnia with Chinese herbs more affordably and without the side effects associated with prescriptions. One study looked at more than 16,000 Taiwanese patients complaining of insomnia who were successfully treated with Chinese herbs. The patients had received a grand total of 29,801 Chinese herbal medicine prescriptions. The data concluded the most common individual Chinese herbs prescribed for insomnia were *Polygonum multiflorum* (used 23.8 percent of the time), followed by *Ziziphus spinosa* (18.3 percent), and *Poria cocos* (13.3 percent).

These are exactly the main ingredients in that lovely little Chinese herb PAC that I discovered at the conference and have been using ever since. The product is called iSleep HerbPac and it's available through PacHerbs (www.pacherbs.com).

Kidney Stones

Use This Combo Cure and Take a Pass on This Painful Condition

I'VE NEVER HAD kidney stones, but I've heard people describe the pain of passing them as akin to pulling your upper lip over the back of your head. (Or maybe that was a description of childbirth.) In any case, no one I know who's ever had them—kidney stones, that is, not kids—is eager to repeat the experience.

Kidney stones are hard masses that can grow from crystals forming within the kidneys. Women get them, but they're much more common in men. About three-quarters of the stones are made out of calcium oxalate. (Uric acid stones are most commonly found in gout.)

Oxalate is an organic salt, but when combined with calcium it produces an insoluble mass called calcium-oxalate, which is the most common chemical compound found in kidney stones. Urinary oxalate is the single strongest predictor of kidney stone formation—the higher the urinary oxalate, the greater the risk of oxalate kidney stones.

So anything that helps reduce urinary oxalate would help reduce the risk of kidney stones, right? That's the finding of a recent and important study in which supplementation with 900 mg EPA and 600 mg DHA for a period of

30 days lowered the urinary oxalate by 23 percent, thus effectively decreasing, by a significant amount the risk of calcium oxalate formation.

Because 75 percent of kidney stones are formed from oxalates, you'll want to avoid or at least reduce your consumption of foods that are high in oxalates: nuts, tea, chocolate, beets, rhubarb, and wheat bran are all on the list. Phosphate-based soft drinks are also a big problem for stone formers. A study in the *Journal of Clinical Epidemiology* examined 1,009 male patients and found that the guys who consumed the largest quantities of phosphate-based sodas had the highest rate of stone recurrence.

Two other things you can you do to help prevent another excruciatingly painful stone from ever forming again is to take magnesium and start drinking a ton of water. Water will make calcium oxalate more soluble and a lot less likely to form crystals. Water and lemon juice may help as well, because a half cup of lemon juice a day will raise citrate levels, which can help fight stone formation. (Soda, on the other hand, does the *opposite*.) And research shows that grapefruit juice raises the risk of stones by as much as 44 percent, so if you're prone to stone formation, avoid it. Ditto with salt.

The Magic of Magnesium

According to Alan Gaby, M.D., author of the textbook *Nutritional Medicine*, research "strongly suggests that supplementing with modest doses of magnesium and vitamin B6 can greatly reduce the recurrence rate of calcium oxalate kidney stones." In one study, 149 patients with long-standing stones received 100 mg of a cheap form of magnesium (magnesium oxide) three times a day, equal to 180 mg per day of elemental magnesium. They also received 10 mg of B6 once a day at the same time.

Would you like to know what happened?

The mean rate of stone formation dropped by 92.3 percent.

Another study published in the *Journal of the American College of Nutrition* showed that supplementing with 500 mg of magnesium a day (even without the B6) dropped stone formation by 90 percent.

"Unfortunately, many doctors remain unaware of this simple, safe, effective, and inexpensive treatment for recurrent kidney stones," Gaby says.

Natural Prescription for Kidney Stones

To reduce recurrences and prevent new calcium oxalate stone formation

Fish oil: 1.5 grams of combined EPA-DHA daily (I recommend Barlean's High Potency EPA-DHA, available at www.jonnybowden.com)

Magnesium citrate: 500 mg

Vitamin B6: 40 mg

Pumpkin seeds: 510 g

Diet: Reduce intake of oxalate-containing foods, increase water and fiber, reduce salt and caffeine. Avoid grapefruit juice.

Low Energy/ Stress Fatigue

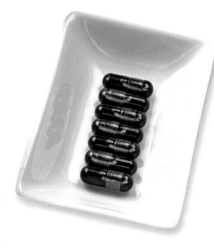

Get a Lift from Rhodiola

IF YOU'RE LOOKING for a natural lift of energy because you've had a rough day, put down the coffee and read on.

Rhodiola is an herb steeped deep in history. Traditionally in Eastern Europe and Asia, rhodiola has been used to stimulate the nervous system, enhance performance, improve sleep, and reduce fatigue. The herb has been included as an official Russian medicine since 1969 and as a Swedish medicine since 1985. Of the 200 Rhodiola species, R. rosea has been studied most extensively, but its properties are not well known in the West because most publications are in Slavic and Scandinavian languages.

Grown primarily in arctic areas of Europe and Asia, rhodiola is categorized as an *adaptogen*. An adaptogen doesn't necessarily move things in one direction; it senses the needs of the system and acts accordingly. Much like the thermostat on your central air conditioning that makes the room warmer if it's too cold and colder if it's too warm, an adaptogen helps protect you by helping your body adapt to physiological stressors. And if you're looking for a natural stress buster, this might be just the ticket.

Firsthand Field Studies

Richard P. Brown, M.D., associate professor of clinical psychiatry at Columbia University College of Physicians and Surgeons in New York, experienced the benefits of R. rosea firsthand when he went with a colleague to northern Mongolia to gather wild R. rosea. They were interested in testing the wild form of R. rosea against domestically grown R. rosea. Brown decided to start taking the herb himself and almost immediately noticed that his mind was sharper, he felt less stressed, and he had more energy.

His wife, Patricia Gerbarg, M.D., also experienced the restorative benefits of R. rosea. Suffering from chronic and debilitating pain and fatigue after being treated for Lyme disease, she started taking R. rosea for its energy-boosting properties. After ten days, her mind was clearer, her concentration was sharper, and her memory was improving.

So from Siberia to Mongolia to Columbia University, the reputation of rhodiola's benefits spread. And there are plenty of studies to back up the folklore. In one study, physicians on night duty received a low dose of R. rosea over

WORTH KNOWING

Rhodiola rosea should be taken early in the day because it can interfere with sleep or cause vivid dreams during the first few weeks of use. It should not be used in patients with bipolar disorder. The herb may have additive effects with other stimulants.

two weeks. At the end of the two weeks there was a significant improvement in the doctors' ability to counteract the effects of fatigue. The tests showed positive results on mental fatigue involving associative thinking, short-term memory, calculation, ability to concentrate, and speed of audiovisual perception.

A Cold War Casualty—Almost

Another study examined R. rosea's effect on the fatigue of Russian students caused by stress during examination periods. One group received R. rosea for twenty days during an examination period, while the other group received a placebo. Their physical and mental performances were assessed before and after the time period, using both objective and subjective criteria. The results? Significant improvement in physical fitness, mental fatigue, and motor skills. The group taking rhodiola also rated its own subjective, general well-being significantly better than the placebo group rated its.

During the Cold War, the Soviets looked for a medicine that could boost energy, improve memory, and enhance performance so they could give their military an edge and improve the stamina and performance of their cosmonauts. Soviet scientists documented a wide range of benefits associated with R. rosea from calming the stress response and increasing energy to enhancing physical and mental performance under stress. According to author Peter Jaret, this "super herb" was very nearly lost to Cold War politics.

Protecting the Brain

Because it is an adaptogen, R. rosea may also protect against all sorts of stressors. A number of studies have shown that R. rosea increases physical work capacity and dramatically shortens the recovery time between periods of high-intensity exercise. Admittedly, some controversy exists over its power to increase physical stamina; more clinical trials are needed, but it's looking promising. And speaking of stressors, it's worth noting that in Middle Asia, R. rosea tea was an effective treatment for cold and flu during severe Asian winters.

Stress, over time, can interfere with memory systems and ultimately cause shrinkage of an important area of the brain called the hippocampus, which is intimately involved with memory. R. rosea's protective effect on neurotransmitters (chemical messengers) in the brain helps to enhance thinking, analyzing, evaluating, calculating, planning, and remembering.

But wait, there's more! R. rosea has effects on the endocrine and reproductive systems. In mountain villages of Siberia, a bouquet of rhodiola roots is still given to couples prior to marriage to enhance fertility and ensure the birth of healthy children. Studies have shown that R. rosea improves amenorrhea (loss of menstrual cycle) in women and sexual dysfunction in men. That alone makes it worth the price of admission!

Natural Prescription for Low Energy/Stress Fatigue

Rhodiola rosea: 100 to 170 mg. Make sure it's an extract of the R. rosea root. This is the most effective and has significant animal and human studies.

Note: All dosages are daily dosages and in pill or capsule form unless otherwise noted.

Macular Degeneration/ Vision Issues

Prevent Eyesight Problems with Antioxidants

Omega-3

Zinc

Multi-Vitamin

Lutein

THERE ARE A LOT of things I don't want to be when I grow older, but one of them is blind. Especially when it's preventable—which, in a huge number of cases, it is.

The leading cause of blindness in adults under the age of sixty is diabetic retinopathy, caused by complications of long-term diabetes. But the leading cause of adult blindness and vision loss in adults over sixty is something called macular degeneration. And a few simple supplements can significantly reduce the risk of your ever getting it.

You may recall from high school biology that the retina contains two types of photoreceptors—cones and rods. Cones are the ones that provide color sensitivity, and most of them are located in the central area of the retina in a structure called the macula. So when the macula "degenerates," you're in trouble—color vision and vision sharpness both deteriorate significantly, and in the worst case scenario, you can be looking at blindness (excuse the pun!).

The cause of macular degeneration is not really known, but it's believed that there is an insufficient disposal of waste materials from the cells. Cell waste is normally carried off, but in this case some is left behind and it blocks the light. Essential vision decreases; you always have peripheral vision, but you lose your central vision. In other words, you can't recognize faces or watch TV.

Risk Factors and Solutions

Macular degeneration affects millions of Americans. Smoking, poor diet, and obesity all increase the risk, as do high blood pressure and a number of factors that you can't control (like family history, aging, and the newly discovered complement factor H (CFH) gene, which is strongly associated with macular degeneration). But what you eat—and the supplements you take—affect the macula, and research shows that diet and supplements can be used to treat or prevent the condition.

In 2001, the National Eye Institute conducted the Age-Related Eye Disease Study (AREDS), which involved more than 3,600 people. Researchers found that supplementation with certain nutrients reduced the risk of progressing to advanced macular degeneration by 25 percent, especially in groups at highest risk. They reported a significant 27 percent reduction in risk for vision loss in these higher-risk groups.

What were those nutrients? A simple antioxidant combo consisting of 500 mg vitamin C, 400 IU vitamin E, 15 mg beta-carotene, and 80 mg zinc.

But there are two important nutrients for the eye that were not included in the study. Why? Because not much was known about them at the time of the research. Not anymore. We now know that *lutein* and *zeaxanthin*—two members of the carotenoid family that are emerging as the superstars of eye nutrition—are vitally important for vision. Lutein and its related compound, zeaxanthin, are highly concentrated in the macula, providing a yellow color known as the macular pigment, which protects the macula. You want that pigment to be dense, the better to protect your eyes.

A 1997 study found that subjects fed a diet high in spinach and corn experienced nearly a 20 percent increase in macular pigment density. What's the connection with those foods? That diet effectively boosted the subjects' consumption of lutein about 400 percent and zeaxanthin about 300 percent. That same year it was found that the use of a lutein supplement can also increase the density of the protective macular pigment. You can, of course, get some lutein from foods such as spinach, kale, broccoli, and Brussels sprouts, though probably not enough to get the full therapeutic effect of supplements.

In 2004, the Lutein Antioxidant Supplementation Trial (LAST) found that subjects receiving lutein or lutein plus antioxidants showed a significant

WORTH KNOWING

Michael Geiger, O.D., a nutritionally minded optometrist and author of *Eye Care Naturally*, also recommends garlic. "Garlic helps with circulation," he told me. "One of the problems with macular degeneration is the buildup of waste products, so you want to get the blood flowing."

increase in macular density and in some measures, visual function. Virtually every expert now includes lutein and zeaxanthin (they are usually found together) in any formula for eye health and for the prevention of macular degeneration and adult vision loss.

The Power of Antioxidants

Both antioxidants and omega-3 fatty acids can help protect your eyes and preserve your vision in a variety of ways.

Oily fish—and the omega-3 fatty acids found in them—can help protect against macular degeneration. A review of omega-3 functions in the retina

Natural Prescription for Preventing Macular Degeneration and Preserving Vision

Multivitamin: Containing at least 500 mg vitamin C, 400 IU vitamin E, and 15 mg beta-carotene

Zinc: 30 to 80 mg

Omega-3 fatty acids: 1,000 mg (1 g)

Lutein (and zeaxanthin): 10 mg for general prevention, 20 to 40 mg for someone who already has macular degeneration

Note: All dosages are daily dosages and in pill or capsule form unless otherwise noted.

from the National Eye Institute's Division of Epidemiology and Clinical Research suggests that omega-3 fatty acids play a pivotal role in protecting the retina. They should be included in any program for eye health and vision preservation. And while you're at it, take a multivitamin. An analysis of data from the Physicians Health Study shows that taking a multivitamin supplement can decrease the risk of cataracts.

Antioxidants protect cells throughout the body, not just in the eyes. And some have multiple effects. Zinc, for example again, is critical for the functioning of the immune system. An interesting and little noted "side effect" of AREDS was that participants who received zinc, either alone or with the other antioxidants, had lower rates of death than those not taking zinc. Hey, an extra few years of healthy life is a nice "side benefit" of taking a few antioxidants that can preserve your vision!

In addition to being an antioxidant, zinc improves the transport and use of cysteine, an amino acid needed to manufacture glutathione, arguably the most important antioxidant in the body.

Interestingly, eye problems can be a predictor of other health issues and even mortality. According to Harvard researcher Johanna Seddon, M.D., sick eyes are especially likely to show up in people who are sick with other illnesses. There's a well-established link between macular degeneration and cardiovascular disease, for example, and the two share a number of risk factors, including obesity, smoking, and inflammation.

Migraines

Ease Your Mind with These Herbs and Nutrients

Willow Bark

Riboflavin B2

Magnesium

CoQ10

5-HTP

Feverfew

WHETHER YOU'VE been hit with a classic low-grade migraine or a full-blown migraine complete with aura and flashing lights, these are the worst type of headaches and can be debilitating for many people.

Not to be confused with tension headaches, migraines are much more severe and incapacitating, lasting anywhere from four to seventy-two hours. More women experience migraines than men, most likely because of the role that hormones play (consider the fact that many women get them either right before or during menstruation and that most migraines actually disappear after menopause).

But there's hope. Research has shown that a number of nutrients—and a couple of powerful herbs—may significantly help sufferers of migraines (and perhaps headaches in general). And it's those nutrients—CoQ10, riboflavin, and magnesium—and herbs—butterbur and feverfew—that form the backbone of the natural prescription for migraines, with maybe some 5-HTP thrown in for good measure. Read on.

How a Migraine Begins

No one really knows for sure what causes a migraine; the triggers can be different and varied for each person. When that switch is flipped on, a series of events takes place within the nerve cells of the brain. Substances called *excitotoxins* overstimulate these nerve cells. They also cause the warning signs that commonly precede a migraine: depression, irritability, restlessness, loss of appetite, and an aura that most describe as brightly colored lights. As this is happening, the nerve cells send out impulses to the brain's blood vessels and release substances that cause inflammation and swelling.

So what causes the nerve cells to get excited in the first place? Truth is, the list is long and varied, and differs from person to person. Some of the usual suspects include anxiety, stress, lack of food, lack of sleep, exposure to light, and hormonal changes in women. And then there are food triggers (more on that in a moment) and the possibility of missing nutrients in the diet. There is even some information that suggests a link to the bacterial infection H. pylori.

One promising line of research suggests that people who are prone to headaches may benefit by supplemental 5-hydroxytryptophan or 5-HTP. 5-HTP is made in the body from the amino acid *tryptophan* and then converted into serotonin, the "feel good" brain chemical. In one study a group of headache sufferers received 300 mg of 5-HTP a day. This group had a significant reduction in their use of painkillers as well as a significant decrease in the number of days with headaches in the two weeks following the study. The patients in this study suffered with chronic tension-type headaches, but there's reason to think 5-HTP might be a useful adjunct for those with migraines as well.

The excellent evidence-based monograph on 5-HTP—written as a collaboration between Natural Standard (www.naturalstandard.com) and the faculty of Harvard Medical School—states that "there is evidence from several studies in both children and adults that 5-HTP may be effective in reducing the severity and frequency of headaches, including tension headaches and migraines. 5-HTP may be most effective for treating headaches in people with a history of depression or those who experienced severe headaches before the age of 20 years."

Diet: Avoiding the Trigger Foods

Then there are food triggers, some of which you might not want to hear about but I'll tell you anyway: chocolate and alcohol come to mind. (Hey, isn't it worth a trial period without them just to see if it helps? It really might.) Maybe it's not chocolate or alcohol—maybe it's salt. It could be sugar. It could be milk. It could be wine. In fact, it could be anything that flips that brain switch and releases those excitotoxins.

And by the way, I didn't pick on chocolate and alcohol just to annoy you—truth is, they're among the most common culprits largely because they contain *tyramines*. Tyramines are chemicals derived from the amino acid *tyrosine*. For many people, tyramines are a huge trigger for migraines. In addition to chocolate and alcoholic beverages, high-tyramine foods include anything fermented (like aged cheeses, fermented soy sauce, and sauerkraut) and processed meats like pepperoni and sausage.

Individuals who have reactive hypoglycemia—low blood sugar that occurs one to three hours after a meal—may find that being on the blood-sugar roller coaster triggers severe headaches. Reducing refined sugar and eating smaller, more frequent meals (with more protein, fat, and fiber) will help balance blood sugar and keep it on a more even keel. But for goodness' sake, don't reach for aspartame instead of sugar: It contains an amino acid called phenylalanine, which also has the potential to be a migraine trigger. (I won't even get into the whole aspartame story—let's not go there. Suffice it to say, I don't recommend it even if you don't suffer from headaches.)

I wish there were an easy formula for determining what your individual triggers are, but there isn't. But make like Columbo and do some good detective work. If you systematically note what triggers, e.g., environmental, food, interpersonal, etc. seem to precipitate an attack, you'll eventually hit pay dirt.

And it's not just the things you're eating (but maybe shouldn't be) that can trigger an attack—it could also be the absence of things in your diet that should be there. (Since we can't know for sure just what those missing ele-

WORTH KNOWING

According to a 1999 study in the *Medical Tribune* about 10 to 15 percent of women who suffer migraines have them primarily during their menstrual cycle. Satisfying carbohydrate cravings before the cycle, eating irregularly, snacking frequently, and poor sleep can increase the risk of menstrual migraines. Regular, moderate exercise helps.

ments might be, the best advice is to make your diet as rich in whole foods, antioxidants, minerals, omega-3 fats, and plant phytochemicals as possible. It's the ultimate "can't hurt, might help!" strategy.)

Now Add in the Combos: Three Nutrients, Two Herbs

Riboflavin (vitamin B2), magnesium, and coenzyme Q10 (CoQ10) have been researched, reviewed, and studied for their effectiveness in managing migraines. They are all good, effective alternative treatments and can help to prevent migraines. CQ10 is a nutrient that is normally associated with energy: It helps the cells use oxygen. Andrew Hershey, M.D., Ph.D., associate director of neurology research at Cincinnati Children's Hospital Medical Center, looked at its relation to migraine in a recent study done at the University of Cincinnati. He examined 1,552 children and adolescents between the ages of three and twenty-two and found that most had insufficient CoQ10 levels. After supplementing with CoQ10, the frequency of headaches fell significantly. Those affected went from having migraines an average of 19.2 days per month to 12.5 days per month. That's a big difference when you are experiencing a migraine, and when you're a teen whose state of mind and feeling of well-being play a big role in determining how successful your social life is.

Another study done in 2005 examined CoQ10's effect on adult migraine sufferers. Those who took 300 mg of CoQ10 for four months experienced a 50 percent or greater reduction in frequency of migraine attacks, significantly different from those just using a placebo. As for side effects in the groups in both of these studies: none.

Riboflavin, or vitamin B2, is another nutrient that has been shown to be effective in the treatment of migraines. It can potentially decrease the number of migraine days by about 25 percent and lower the frequency by 30 percent. Similar to CoQ10, riboflavin is needed to convert food into energy. Dairy products, eggs, and meat contain significant amounts of B2 but wouldn't come close to providing the high doses you would need to treat a migraine. Remember that all the B vitamins work synergistically; when taking any single B vitamin therapeutically, it's best to also take a B-complex vitamin as a base and then, at a different time of day, add that extra therapeutic dose of B2.

Magnesium also plays an important role in migraine prevention and reduction. Like 5-HTP, it has an effect on serotonin, so when magnesium levels are low, the risk for a migraine may increase. Magnesium also improves energy production in the heart, plus it dilates the arteries, helping blood deliver oxygen more effectively. Up to 50 percent of patients who experience acute migraines have been shown to have a magnesium deficiency. This is actually not surprising because most adults in the United States—75 percent by some estimates—are deficient in this important mineral. The National Academy of Sciences recommends that all women over the age of thirty take 320 mg of magnesium daily, but half of them consume only 230 mg or even less. The academy suggests more for men: 420 mg, yet only half of men over thirty get more than 330 mg.

Beneficial Herbs

Two herbs stand out when it comes to treating migraines: butterbur (Petasites hybridus) and feverfew (Tanacetum parthenium). Compelling evidence from

Natural Prescription for Migraines

CoQ10

Children/Adolescents: 1 to 3 mg per kg of body weight per day in a single dose. Liquid gels are best.

Adults: 100 mg per day, three times daily

Magnesium: 200 to 600 mg

Vitamin B2 (riboflavin): 400 mg per day for three months. Take in addition to a B-complex supplement.

5-HTP: 200 to 600 mg

Butterbar: 100 to 150 mg;

Feverfew: 300 mg, twice daily for 12 weeks;

White Willow Bark: (300 mg, twice daily for 12 weeks)

Diet: Avoid refined sugar, alcohol, caffeine, aspartame, smoking, salt, and tyramine-containing foods

Reduce stress and get enough sleep

Check for food allergies

Note: The dosages are daily and in pill or capsule form unless otherwise noted.

human trials suggests that butterbur may have real benefits in preventing migraines. One hundred and eight children and adolescents between the ages of six and seventeen tried butterbur root extract for four months and experienced a decrease in the frequency of migraine attacks. In addition, they all reported feeling better.

The same results were found in adults. In one study, Pedadolex—a patented, high-quality butterbur preparation that you can buy in stores—was used at the dosage of 25 mg twice daily for twelve weeks. The frequency of migraine attacks decreased by a whopping 60 percent—and no side effects were reported to boot.

The most frequently used herb for the long-term prevention of migraines is feverfew. A number of well-done studies have suggested that feverfew may prevent migraine headaches. In studies, feverfew users seem to have milder headaches, fewer headaches, and less vomiting and nausea (though the herb doesn't necessarily shorten the length of time each headache lasts). Using feverfew together with another herb, white willow bark, also reduces the frequency, intensity, and duration of migraine attacks, by up to 60 percent.

Polycystic Ovary Syndrome (PCOS)

Attack These Symptoms with a Low-Carb Diet

WHEN I HEAR the three words "polycystic ovary syndrome (PCOS)," the first thing I think of is insulin resistance. And the next thing I think of is a low-carb diet. Let me explain. PCOS is both a metabolic and a hormonal disorder. No one knows exactly what causes it, but there are a number of risk factors (see below). As the name suggests, it's a syndrome, which means it's more like a collection of multiple symptoms than an actual disease. Many doctors who see women with these symptoms don't necessarily connect the dots, and many women seek treatment for the individual symptoms from specialists who may miss the larger picture.

It can go completely undiagnosed because its symptoms overlap with so many other health concerns. Many women—and their doctors—wind up treating the symptoms of PCOS, such as acne or infertility, as separate and discrete problems. They'll go to a dermatologist about their acne, for example, and call it a day, never suspecting that the acne is just a symptom of a whole underlying process.

The result? Many women who have PCOS don't actually know it.

The Insulin Connection

One thing that almost always goes with PCOS is weight gain, and women with PCOS find it fiendishly difficult to lose weight, even with dieting and exercise. One thing we know for sure is that women with PCOS are much more likely to have a condition called insulin resistance, which is also associated with metabolic syndrome and type 2 diabetes. Our diet can significantly aggravate the condition of insulin resistance, which is why dietary intervention can be so effective in all conditions where it is a problem.

A low-carb diet is the absolute best strategy for dealing with PCOS naturally. According to many experts, one of the biggest contributors to PCOS is poor diet, especially a high intake of refined carbohydrates. Because insulin resistance is such a huge contributor to the PCOS, a diet that helps control blood sugar and insulin is the first order of business. Too much sugar, or foods that convert quickly into sugar like potatoes and starches, causes a rise in insulin, a hormone that not only aggravates PCOS but also contributes to weight gain.

The weight gain–PCOS links is a classic chicken-and-egg dilemma. We're not sure whether women get PCOS because they are overweight (or obese) or whether they become overweight (or obese) because they have PCOS in the first place. We do know, however, that the two are intimately connected. Fifty percent of women with PCOS are overweight.

Do You Have PCOS?

No single blood test can determine whether you have PCOS, so it takes a bit of detective work to identify what's really going on. It's estimated that

5 to 10 percent of women of childbearing age have PCOS. Some of the symptoms include:

- **Menstrual irregularities:** infrequent periods, no periods, or irregular bleeding
- **Infertility or the inability to get pregnant due to not ovulating**
- **Facial hair (or hair on chest, stomach, back, thumbs, or toes)**
- **Acne**
- **Weight gain or obesity**
- **Thinning hair (or male pattern hair loss)**

PCOS sufferers have an increased risk for some very serious diseases. Later in life, women with PCOS are at higher risk for developing type 2 diabetes, high blood pressure, heart disease, and cancer.

Ovarian Cysts

As the name of the disorder suggests, women with PCOS frequently have many ovarian cysts. The cysts don't necessarily rupture, but if they do it can be agonizing, even though it's not necessarily medically dangerous.

Each month the ovaries cause a number of follicles to ripen. These follicles are actually cysts, pockets of tissue filled with fluid and hormones (mostly estrogen). Normally, one (or two) of these follicles become dominant and actually produce an egg. The egg pops out of the follicle and goes into the fallopian tube, which in turn triggers a whole bunch of hormonal events such as the secretion of progesterone that in turn will help support a pregnancy if the egg is fertilized. In this "normal" scenario, the egg becomes a little factory (the corpus luteum) for making progesterone, and the concentration of progesterone in the body can become a couple of hundred times higher than estrogen. That's normal. If there's no fertilization, the "factory" stops its hormonal production of estrogen and progesterone and the uterine lining sheds, resulting in a menstrual period. The low levels of hormones then cause the cycle to begin all over again.

But with PCOS, a lot of follicles are created but no one follicle becomes predominant. Ovulation is disrupted, making it very difficult to get pregnant. (Women with PCOS have a 10 to 15 percent greater risk of miscarriage than women without it.) Estrogen becomes dominant and isn't balanced by sufficient progesterone, and other hormones, called androgens, remain high. The result is a host of symptoms, triggered by or aggravated by a hormonal imbalance characterized by elevated levels of male hormones and low levels of progesterone.

These hormonal imbalances prevent ovulation from taking place regularly and cause the ovaries to form multiple cysts. Adding to the difficulty in identifying the underlying problem is the fact that 30 percent of women with PCOS don't actually present with cysts.

Enter insulin.

A Low-Carb Diet Is the Answer

High-carbohydrate diets stimulate high blood sugar, which in turn stimulates high levels of insulin, especially in susceptible people. High levels of insulin then stimulate the androgen receptors on the outside of the ovary, which may lead to more cysts as well as other problems related to too much androgen production. And high insulin levels are thought to increase the production of male hormones. Thus high levels of insulin are intimately connected to the typical PCOS symptoms of excess facial hair, thin hair on the head, and acne. The high level of insulin also further increases the risk of obesity. Bringing down insulin (and the blood sugar that drives it up) becomes a priority.

When we speak of insulin resistance, we tend to forget that not all tissues and cells become resistant at the same time. In fact, some don't become resistant at all. For example, overweight people may—at least in the beginning—have very nonresistant fat cells. In fact, far from being resistant to its siren call, their fat cells may just love insulin and sugar. Their muscle cells may refuse to take any more sugar, but the fat cells say, "Hey, bring it on!" These fat cells are said to be insulin sensitive.

And guess what? The ovaries also tend to remain insulin sensitive. That means that if there's a genetic predisposition for the ovaries to overproduce androgen hormones—as there is with women who have PCOS—the excess insulin that's sent into the bloodstream to deal with the excess sugar winds up bathing these nonresistant tissues in an ocean of insulin that's way too much for their needs. And one of the responses to all that insulin hitting the ovaries is that they produce even more testosterone and androstenedione, which leads to hair loss, acne, obesity, infertility, and other symptoms of PCOS.

Enter the low-carb diet, the perfect "natural" solution to high levels of insulin and to the problem of insulin resistance.

Conventional Medicine: An Incomplete Answer

Conventional medicine usually treats PCOS with drugs that lower levels of male hormones (androgens) or with diabetes medications that help the body to utilize insulin better. For women who don't want to become pregnant, docs will sometimes use birth control pills to help regulate menstrual cycles, clear up acne, and reduce levels of male hormones, but the Pill does not cure PCOS.

Metformin, a drug known by its trade name of Glucophage, is often given to people with diabetes or metabolic syndrome because it helps the body utilize insulin more effectively. Research published in the *British Medical Journal* and elsewhere shows that metformin is effective in helping women with PCOS achieve ovulation, and it reduces insulin concentrations and blood pressure as well. It also helps patients lose weight. On the other hand, it's also associated with a higher incidence of nausea, vomiting, and other gastrointestinal disturbance. That said, it might be helpful.

WORTH KNOWING

Stress can elevate hormones that in turn contribute to excessive insulin and blood sugar. Biofeedback, stress reduction, and meditation have been shown to reduce a hormone that stimulates many of the physiological processes that can aggravate or contribute to PCOS. Depression frequently accompanies PCOS, perhaps because good mood is one of the serious casualties of hormone imbalances. Consider meditation or any other stress-reducing technique as well as exercise, which elevates mood, as important natural components of any treatment plan for PCOS.

Biotin and Fenugreek

Yet many experts consider it something of a Band-Aid on the problem, which doesn't get to the cause of PCOS. Remember that the main thing metformin does is help the body use insulin better. Chromium picolinate does the same thing and is a great supplement to use together with a low-carb diet to help manage both blood sugar and insulin.

In addition to chromium, which improves glucose tolerance, decreases fasting blood sugar, and has been shown to help insulin resistance in people with diabetes, two other supplements may be helpful. Though not normally thought of as the first nutrient you'd take for PCOS, biotin in high doses (8 to 16 mg) should be considered because it has the potential to be of great help in normalizing and lowering blood sugar.

And then there's fenugreek, an herb that also has a beneficial effect on blood sugar. It reduces fasting blood glucose (blood sugar) when used at the dosage of 1.5 to 2 mg per kg of body weight. (Note: Just to be on the safe side, I wouldn't use fenugreek while pregnant; be aware of this, since many people may first discover they have PCOS while trying to conceive.)

Weight Loss: Slow but Successful

The single most effective thing you can do to help the symptoms of PCOS is to lose weight. Some research shows that it really doesn't matter what kind of diet you use to accomplish this—high protein, low protein, etc.—but losing weight absolutely helps normalize the symptoms of PCOS.

Most holistic or complementary health practitioners favor a low-carb (or low-glycemic) diet for anyone who has blood sugar or insulin problems. That means high-quality protein, good fats, such as olive oil, coconut oil, some butter, avocado, flaxseed oil, fish oil, and nuts, and some low-sugar fruits, such as grapefruit and berries. Get the sugar out of your diet and reduce calories, something that will be a lot easier to do on a higher-protein, lower-carbohydrate diet.

It's just way easier to manage blood sugar and bring down insulin levels with a diet higher in protein, fiber from vegetables, and good fats than it is on a diet high in refined carbs, flour, and sugar, even if it's lower in calories.

Keep in mind, however, that weight loss for an individual with PCOS may be slower than weight loss for someone without the condition. It will take time for your metabolism to "heal itself" before the weight comes off. So be patient and stay committed to a healthy diet for the long haul.

Natural Prescription for Polycystic Ovary Syndrome

Low-carb (low-glycemic) diet

GOES WELL WITH:

Chromium picolinate or polynicotinate:
1,000 mcg

Biotin: 8 to 16 mg

Note: All dosages are daily dosages and in pill or capsule form unless otherwise noted.

Post-Traumatic Stress Disorder/ Trauma

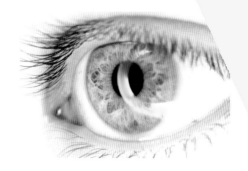

Use EMDR to Help

EMDR, or eye movement desensitization and reprocessing, is a highly regarded, well-researched form of therapy for trauma and post-traumatic stress disorder (PTSD).

It's even gained the respect of the American Psychiatric Association, which found it to have "robust empirical support and demonstrated effectiveness." In its 2004 edition of *Practice Guideline for the Treatment of Patients with Acute Stress Disorder and Post-Traumatic Stress Disorder*, the association gave EMDR therapy its "highest level of recommendation" for the treatment of trauma. And if that's not enough, the Department of Veterans Affairs' and the Department of Defense's 2004 Clinical Practice Guideline for the Management of Post-Traumatic Stress placed EMDR in the "A" category as "strongly recommended" for the treatment of trauma.

The originator and developer of the therapy is Francine Shapiro, Ph.D., a senior research fellow at the Mental Research Institute in Palo Alto, California, and a recipient of the Distinguished Scientific Achievement in Psychology Award presented by the California Psychological Association.

Back in 1987, while walking in the park and thinking about some personal distressing memories, she happened to notice that eye movements appeared to decrease the negative emotions associated with them. Like many great innovators in healing (or in science, for that matter), she expanded on what was essentially a fortuitous personal discovery, began experimenting, developed a theory, put it to the test, and eventually developed the treatment approach that is now EMDR.

So what the heck is it?

When Trauma Happens

As noted above, EMDR stands for eye movement desensitization and reprocessing, and it's based on a theory about the way we process information. The theory, simplified, is this: We humans all have a built-in data processing system that takes all the multiple elements of experience and integrates them. These "memory networks" contain thoughts, images, associations, emotions, and sensations. So, for example, you might have an experience of learning to ride a bicycle that involves visual information, sensory information, data (time, place, and year), and emotions (it was thrilling, it was scary, I felt powerful, I felt helpless, etc.).

Shapiro sees the brain's information processing network as analogous to other body systems like digestion, where food goes in and gets "processed," and the gut extracts nutrients for health and survival. If something interferes with food being wholly "processed" in your body, any number of things can result, from an upset stomach to a food sensitivity to—in a severe case of allergy—anaphylactic shock.

The strong negative feelings may very well interfere with the normal information processing that would otherwise take place when trauma occurs, according to Shapiro. And if the information related to a distressing or traumatic experience isn't fully processed by the brain's central processing mechanism, the initial perceptions, emotions, and distorted thoughts will be "undigested"—they'll be stored exactly as they were first experienced at the time of the event, and you may well relive them every time a memory is triggered.

So let's take, for example, a rape victim.

A rape survivor may very well know intellectually that the attack wasn't her fault, but this information may not override or connect with her feeling that she somehow brought the attack on herself. The memory is then stored "dysfunctionally," without the appropriate connections, much like food that hasn't been processed by the right digestive enzymes. When she thinks about

WORTH KNOWING

The EMDR Humanitarian Assistance Program (HAP) is a nonprofit that has been described as a kind of mental health equivalent of Doctors Without Borders. It's a global network of clinicians who travel anywhere there is a need to stop suffering and prevent the aftereffects of trauma and violence. Its trauma recovery network coordinates clinicians to treat victims and emergency service workers after such crises as Hurricane Katrina and the 9/11 attacks. For more information, go to www.emdrhap.org.

the trauma—or when a memory of it is triggered by some situation or image or thought—she may feel like she is reliving it. This is pretty much a definition of what happens in post-traumatic stress disorder.

How EMDR Therapy Helps

So what happens in therapy? At the heart of EMDR is what's called dual attention stimulus. Most commonly, the therapist will ask you to mentally focus on the distressing (or desired) experience while at the same time directing your attention to an external stimulus (most commonly eye movements, though auditory tones or even tapping can be used as well). It's believed that this dual attention phenomena helps facilitate information processing and helps the trauma survivor integrate the elements of the experience in order to deal with them.

While the various theories that have been proposed to explain why EMDR works are dense and laden with terminology from neurobiology, a simple version is that humans have what's called an orienting response hardwired into our brains. We pay attention to what moves: It served us well from an evolutionary perspective, else our caveman ancestors would not have recognized danger in the woods. (The orienting response could also be seen as a kind of investigatory reflex, the brain's way of saying, "What the heck is this?" You can see a demonstration of this phenomenon by playing peek-a-boo with any infant!)

It's been suggested that the orienting response somehow disrupts the traumatic memory network and interrupts previous associations to negative emotions. It's also been suggested that the investigatory reflex itself is like a psychic deep breathing in that it results in a basic relaxation response. None of these theories are mutually exclusive.

Whatever the underlying neurobiology, the treatment works. An enormous amount of research has validated its ability to help people with trauma and PTSD deal with their issues so that previously disturbing memories (and present situations that trigger them) are no longer debilitating and new healthy responses can emerge. Two separate studies have indicated an elimination of the diagnosis of PTSD in 83 to 90 percent of civilian participants after four to seven sessions, and many others have found a significant decrease in a wide range of symptoms after three or four sessions.

My friend Daniel Amen, M.D., a psychiatrist, brain imaging specialist, and professor of psychiatry at the University of California, has been taking SPECT scans (brain pictures) of his patients and using EMDR with post-traumatic stress patients. He's reported a decrease in the activity of the anterior cingulate, basal ganglia, and deep limbic areas, all sections of the brain deeply involved in emotions, trauma, and memories.

By the way, it's not just major traumatic events—or what EMDR therapists call "large-T traumas"—that can cause psychological distress. It can even be a (relatively) small event like being bullied or teased. As we all know, even these seemingly small experiences can leave lasting imprints and still have the power to elicit powerful emotions years or even decades later. EMDR can help with these as well.

EMDR is not a one-session "cure," but rather an eight-phase process in which the EMDR-trained psychiatrist or psychotherapist may integrate other effective psychotherapy protocols ranging from cognitive behavioral therapies to body-centered approaches. It's not necessarily effective for every condition, nor does it claim to be. But it positively shines in the area of trauma and

PTSD. At a recent seminar I attended on the brain given by Amen and largely attended by therapists, I met more than one practitioner who said to me, "I'd never recommend a therapist for post traumatic stress disorder who didn't incorporate EMDR in [his or her] treatment."

PMS

Feel Better Each Month with Dr. Jonny's PMS Cocktail

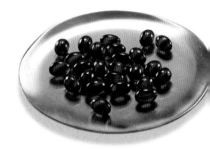

AS ANYONE WHO has experienced it knows well, PMS is no picnic. It's also—let me be very clear—*not* "all in your head." It's the product of a real hormonal turbulence that accompanies the menstrual cycle, more in some people than in others, and it can cause significant mood swings, crying jags, depression, anger, and irritability, not to mention a compendium of physical symptoms like bloat, constipation, and terrible cramps.

That hormonal storm, which can be a light tropical rain for some folks and Hurricane Katrina for others, also affects neurotransmitters like serotonin, influencing mood, cravings, and behavior. The combination of nutrients I'm about to tell you about works wonders.

The Dynamic Duo: Magnesium and Vitamin B6

Let's start with magnesium. Supplementation with magnesium can improve mood and also help with fluid retention.

In one of many studies, supplementation with 360 mg of magnesium three times a day (just a little more than the amount in my recommended PMS cocktail) produced significantly improved scores on the Moos Menstrual Distress Questionnaire, leading the researchers to conclude that magnesium supplementation could represent an effective treatment of premenstrual symptoms related to mood changes.

Vitamin B6 has long been observed to be part of a comprehensive nutritional support package for PMS. The body needs B6 to make serotonin out of the amino acid *tryptophan*, and many people are low in B6 (as well as other B vitamins) because of stress, which literally eats up B vitamins for breakfast! And who couldn't use more relaxing, calming, crave-busting serotonin? Research shows that supplementing with B6 up to 100 mg a day is very likely to be of benefit in treating premenstrual symptoms and premenstrual depression.

One study in the *Journal of Women's Health and Gender-Based Medicine* tested various combinations of B6 and magnesium and found that both B6 and the B6-magnesium combo were helpful in reducing mild PMS-related anxiety symptoms. This study was all the more interesting because they used a crappy kind of magnesium—magnesium oxide—and a low dose to boot, but folks still reported improvements. A high-quality magnesium at the 800 mg dose I recommend, together with B6, would be likely to produce even better results.

Using the Right Dose of Evening Primrose Oil

Evening primrose oil (like borage oil and black currant oil) is a natural source of a fatty acid called GLA—gamma-linolenic acid. This is one of those supplements for PMS that thousands swear by but is lacking in good scientific research that shows that it works. That may be because most of the studies on it used a preparation that contained only 40 mg of GLA, which is too low to have any real effect on PMS symptoms.

The average 1,000 mg dose of evening primrose oil contains about 100 mg of GLA. My "cocktail" would provide at least 200 mg (if not more) of GLA a day. It may also be true that GLA works best in combination with B6 and magnesium and is not quite as effective on its own. Because GLA is a natural anti-inflammatory, and because many people find it helpful for PMS, I think you should include it in the cocktail.

What about Calcium?

There is good scientific evidence for the use of calcium in easing PMS. A lot of research suggests that calcium and vitamin D supplements may reduce the severity of PMS, and there appears to be a link between PMS and low dietary calcium intake. Taking 1 to 1.2 g of calcium daily seems to really reduce depressed mood, water retention, and pain.

In one study, women consuming an average of 1,283 mg of calcium a day from foods had about a 30 percent lower risk of developing PMS compared to women consuming much less (529 mg). A more recent study, in the Archives of Internal Medicine, saw a 40 percent lower risk of PMS developing in women with high intakes of vitamin D and calcium. Considering all the other great things vitamin D does—such as its role in cancer prevention and bone health—and considering that most of us get far too little of it, vitamin D supplements are a good idea.

Remember, if you want to increase your calcium intake, dairy is hardly the only way to do it, though the dairy industry would have you believe it is the best way. It's not. Adding more dairy to your diet opens up a whole other can of worms that you may not want to open (see the section on dairy in my book *The 150 Healthiest Foods on Earth*), and it may even aggravate PMS symptoms. Green leafy vegetables, sardines, and seeds (such as sesame or pumpkin) are full of calcium, and there are always supplements (be sure to take magnesium at the same time).

Neptune Krill Oil

Krill are little crustaceans that look like shrimp and provide food for everything from salmon to blue whales. Their oil is rich in omega-3s, antioxidants, and vitamins; there's good evidence that krill oil can help reduce the symptoms of PMS.

In a double-blind, randomized clinical trial, seventy patients diagnosed with PMS (using the standards of the *Diagnostic and Statistical Manual of Mental Disorders*, third edition, revised) were treated for three months with either krill oil or plain old omega-3 fish oil. The krill oil group had a statistically significant improvement in dysmenorrhea (painful menstruation) as well as in the emotional symptoms of PMS. The women taking the krill oil also chose to consume significantly less painkillers during the treatment period. JMS Medical Research, the independent research organization responsible for the data analysis, reported that krill oil "significantly improves the overall emotional and physical symptoms of patients suffering from premenstrual syndrome."

This study was particularly interesting because it not only investigated the effect of krill oil on PMS, but it also compared the effect of krill oil to regular omega-3 fish oil. Krill oil won. You'd expect omega-3s in general to have a good effect because of their anti-inflammatory action, but possibly other components in the krill oil work synergistically with the omega-3s.

The dose of krill oil found to be most effective is 3 grams a day. The single downside: Neptune Krill Oil is expensive.

Other Helpful Nutrients

The herb chasteberry (vitex) has been used for more than 2,500 years in Egypt, Greece, and Rome for a variety of conditions, not the least of which was decreasing libido (making it popular among celibate clergy but kind of a drag for the rest of those folks). It's widely prescribed in Germany, where the esteemed German Commission E approves it for irregularities of the menstrual cycle and PMS.

Taurine, an amino acid, is a natural diuretic and the best way I know to reduce bloat. One product I use (available through my website) is called Water Ease, and it's almost pure taurine (with a little B6 thrown in for good measure). For water retention I recommend 900 to 1,000 mg of taurine when needed.

And don't forget diet: A great deal of research supports the idea that diet can profoundly affect PMS symptoms. Coffee and alcohol may make things worse. Sugar almost certainly does. Tory Hudson, N.D., a highly respected expert in the field of women's health, wisely recommends a diet of fruits, vegetables, whole grains, legumes, nuts, seeds, and fish, and the avoidance of refined sugar, dairy, salt, tobacco, and caffeine. It might be hard to follow, but it's sure to work.

Natural Prescription for PMS: Dr. Jonny's "PMS Cocktail"

Vitamin B6: 50 mg, twice a day

Magnesium: 400 mg, twice a day

Evening primrose oil: 2,000 mg, twice a day

(or GLA, 320 mg, twice a day)

ALSO WORTH TRYING:

Calcium: 1 to 1.2 grams daily from food and supplements

Neptune Krill Oil: 3 g daily

Taurine (for bloat): 1,000 mg daily

Vitex (herb), also known as chasteberry: Use as directed on label or as instructed by a health practitioner. Studies have used anywhere from about 4 mg per day of the dried extract all the way up to 1,800 mg per day of the dried fruit (in three divided 600 mg doses).

Note: All dosages are daily dosages and in pill or capsule form unless otherwise noted.

Ulcers

Heal Your Stomach with Zinc Carosine

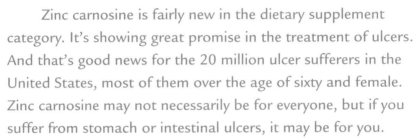

WHAT DO YOU GET when you cross the mineral zinc with the amino acid *carnosine*? The answer may be your ticket to the end of stomach worries.

Zinc carnosine is fairly new in the dietary supplement category. It's showing great promise in the treatment of ulcers. And that's good news for the 20 million ulcer sufferers in the United States, most of them over the age of sixty and female. Zinc carnosine may not necessarily be for everyone, but if you suffer from stomach or intestinal ulcers, it may be for you.

Ulcers start as an irritation in the lining of the stomach wall, which if left untreated, can cause perforations and the all-too-familiar symptoms of heartburn, stomach pain, nausea, and even vomiting. And what do you normally do when this happens?

Plop, Plop, Fizz, Fizz

Well, if you're like millions of Americans, you turn to drugs. Prevacid and Nexium are among the five top-selling prescription drugs in the country, and millions of people use such over-the-counter acid-suppressing drugs as Tums, Maalox, Rolaids, and Mylanta on a daily basis. This is a really bad idea. Over time those antacids do more harm than good.

The only way to get nutrients that our bodies need to function is through digestion, and without the right amount of stomach acid, trying to digest your food and absorb your nutrients is like trying to box with one hand tied behind your back. The major enzyme in the stomach responsible for much of the work of digestion is called pepsin. It's the stomach's principle protein-digesting enzyme, and it requires acid to get "turned on" so it can do its work. Turn off the acid with pills, and pepsin is incapacitated, along with your digestive process.

"Chronic use of antacids may permanently impair normal stomach function," says my friend, naturopathic physician Andrew Rubman, N.D. Some antacids will cause your stomach to produce more acid, a condition called *acid rebound* (or reflux), which worsens your gastrointestinal problem. And some health practitioners believe that overuse of antacids will change the acid-alkaline balance in the gut, upsetting the balance between "good" and "bad" bacteria and setting the stage for infection with *Helicobacter pylori* (*H. pylori*), a common stomach bacterial infection that is a major cause of stomach ulcers.

So antacids are not the answer, not to heartburn and certainly not to ulcers. But zinc carnosine might be. Zinc carnosine dissolves in the stomach and adheres to the ulceration (or wound) on the stomach lining, and it does this more effectively than any other form of zinc. Once dissolved, zinc carnosine goes to work stabilizing membranes, healing wounds, and repairing tissues, all in an effort to support the mucosal barrier—the defensive wall of the stomach.

The Japanese have been using zinc carnosine since 1994 and, in a number of studies, have produced "remarkable improvement" of ulcer symptoms, including heartburn, belching, and abdominal distention.

Gut Science

But the goal here is not just to suppress symptoms—it's to get to the cause of the ulcer in the first place. And that's where zinc carnosine really shines. The two major causes of ulcers are *H. pylori* and nonsteroidal anti-inflammatory drugs (NSAIDs). *H. pylori* affects about 20 percent of adults in the United States. It's found in 70 to 75 percent of gastric ulcer patients and 90 to 100 percent of duodenal ulcer patients. A new study in *Alimentary Pharmacology & Therapeutics* showed that taking antibiotics to kill H. pylori, along with medication to control stomach acid, has an 86 percent success rate, but when zinc carnosine is added to the mix, the success rate climbs to a perfect 100 percent.

NSAIDs, which also include pain relievers such as aspirin and aspirin-like compounds like ibuprofen and naproxen sodium, aren't as innocuous as they seem. They come with their own set of potential side effects, one of which is that they can increase what's called gut *permeability*—essentially a weakening of the lining in the gut that serves as a protective barrier for the bloodstream, keeping out things that don't belong. When those "borders" are weakened, i.e., when the gut becomes more permeable, all manner of digestive "riffraff" can get in, causing myriad health problems. (This is known as *leaky gut* in integrative medicine.)

NSAIDs can complicate the issue. And they've also been linked directly to ulcers. While NSAIDS don't "cause" ulcers, it has been reported that 50 percent of patients who regularly take NSAIDs have some level of gastric erosion and as many as 15 to 30 percent have ulcers.

In early 2007, researchers at the Queen Mary's School of Medicine and Dentistry conducted a series of studies to determine whether zinc carnosine would help protect against the gut-eroding effects of the NSAID drug indomethacin. They treated volunteers with 150 mg of indomethacin every day for five days. But along with their NSAID, half the volunteers also received 75 mg of zinc carnosine a day. The other half of the volunteers received a placebo. Here's what happened: In the NSAID/ placebo group, there was a

Natural Prescription for Ulcers

Zinc carnosine: 75 mg in divided doses. Use for eight weeks to see results

Probiotics: 1 to 10 billion bacteria

Glutamine: 1 to 20 g per day in divided doses

Aloe vera juice: 5 to 30 ml, two or three times per day

Deglycyrrhizinated licorice (DGL) powder: 200 to 400 mg dissolved in 200 ml warm water

Cabbage juice: One quart fresh juice per day. Start slowly and work up to that amount gradually to avoid stomach upset.

Note: All dosages are daily dosages and in pill or capsule form unless otherwise noted.

threefold rise in gut permeability. But in the NSAID group that also received the zinc carnosine, there was virtually none.

The researchers were convinced that zinc carnosine protected the gut against the damages that would have been done by NSAIDs alone, meaning that if you are going to use NSAIDs, taking zinc carnosine at the same time is a really good idea. (An even better idea would be to try zinc carnosine as part of a natural prescription for healing and dump NSAIDs altogether, at least the regular and extended use of them.)

In addition to protecting the intestines, zinc carnosine may help with wound healing in general. In the above-mentioned study, zinc carnosine was found to decrease gastric and small intestinal injury in addition to protecting against gut permeability. Researchers have also found that zinc carnosine encourages cells to travel to a simulated wound area and trigger increased cell proliferation, suggesting that zinc carnosine improves wound healing.

Weight Loss

Burn Fat Faster with Interval Training

THE BEST WORKOUT for burning fat is something called interval training. Interval training is nothing more than the incorporation of short bursts of high-intensity exercise (intervals) into your regular workout.

It's easy to do. If you're walking for an hour, try interspersing short 30 second runs every few minutes. If you're already running, try sprinting faster for 30 seconds. The idea is to alternate these "intervals" of super-hard exercise with more moderate exercise (called "active rest"), during which you catch your breath and get ready to repeat the whole process.

Interval training allows you to maximize the results of your workout, lose more fat, and get fitter, all at the same time. There's no more powerful type of exercise for fat loss on the planet.

Research on interval training and its benefits for both aerobic fitness and fat loss have been going on for decades, but one of the most recent studies was done by an exercise physiologist at the University of Guelph in Ontario, Canada, named Jason Talanian.

"We've always assumed that if you're not too fit you should just get on the bike and go for an hour," Talanian told me in an interview. "But our research has shown really powerful improvements in overall fitness and in fat burning when you increase the intensity for specific intervals."

Doing these spurts of high-intensity exercise leads to physiological adaptations that literally help us burn fat. Specific enzymes in the mitochondria—the powerhouse energy-burning factory in the cell nucleus—become more active through this kind of training. These enzymes—specifically, citrate cynthase and beta-hydroxyacyl-CoA dehydrogenase—break larger fatty acids down into smaller ones.

"This makes it easier to actually burn fat," Talanian says. Besides actual fat burning, measures of cardiovascular fitness—such as maximum oxygen capacity (known as VO2 max)—also improve significantly with this kind of training.

The Research Doesn't Lie!

In Talanian's study, published in the April 2007 *Journal of Applied Physiology*, eight university-age women worked out in his laboratory every other day for two weeks, for a total of seven sessions. During each workout, they performed ten high-intensity intervals of four minutes each. In between each interval they would have two minutes of rest time.

The women were all over the map when it came to fitness levels. Some were completely sedentary, but one was a triathlete and another was a competitive soccer player. The rest were of average fitness and had been exercising in a conventional manner prior to the study (three times a week or so, moderate intensity, kind of what I normally see at the local gym).

"Regardless of their beginning fitness level, all were able to complete at least seven of the ten intervals," Talanian told me. "It was completely doable. And in all subjects we saw increases in the (structures) that escort the fat into the mitochondria where [it] can be burned for energy."

Talanian's study was unusual in that the "high-intensity" intervals were quite long—four minutes each. In previous studies, the "hard" intervals were typically thirty seconds, followed by a lower-intensity, active rest period of two to three minutes. So, for example, if you were walking, you'd speed walk (or run) for your thirty-second interval, and then continue walking (active rest) for two to three minutes while your heart rate slowed a bit. You could repeat that sequence up to ten times per workout.

Talanian hypothesized that one of the reasons for the impressive results in his study was indeed the longer interval of high-intensity work. "I think it's possible that the aerobic component—the last two minutes of the interval—has a lot to do with why we're seeing such adaptations in fat burning."

If four-minute intervals of high intensity seem daunting to you, don't despair. You can get the benefits of interval training with much shorter intervals. One earlier study at McMaster University in Ontario, Canada, found that only four to seven "all-out" bouts of thirty seconds each, alternating with a full, four-minute "recovery" period, still doubled the endurance capacity of the subjects in a mere two weeks of training.

Talanian suggests starting your interval training by computing your maximum heart rate (220 minus your age) and then shooting for a high-intensity interval of 80 percent of that maximum. (You can, of course, work up to that, and you can also start with shorter intervals and increase to longer ones as you improve.)

Most people can't sustain high-intensity exercise for long periods of time. However, we can easily sustain it for thirty seconds to four minutes. By mixing those "high-intensity" intervals into the workout, we're increasing the number of calories burned for the same amount of time.

The PACE Program

One of my favorite docs in the country, Al Sears, M.D., C.N.S., has written an entire program based on fat loss through interval training. It's called PACE (Progressively Accelerating Cardiopulmonary Exertion—a fancy way of saying interval training). Sears—a bit of a contrarian, but a brilliant one—goes so far as to call what most people call "cardio" exercise a waste of time. He believes that forced, continuous endurance exercise induces your heart and lungs to "downsize" because smaller organs allow you to go further, more efficiently, with less rest and less fuel. What's wrong with that, you might ask?

"Instead of building heart strength, (long, slow endurance exercise) robs (the heart) of vital reserve capacity. Heart attacks don't occur because of a lack of endurance. They occur when there is a sudden increase in cardiac demand

WORTH KNOWING

If you're wondering whether you can truly get fit in 12 minutes a week doing interval training properly, the answer is yes. There's a machine called the Xiser invented by an exercise physiologist named Mark J. Smith, Ph.D., and it can get you in better shape than you've ever been in your life if you follow the program exactly as prescribed. It takes about four minutes a day, spread out so that you do one minute at four different times, three times a week, and you're good to go.

If it sounds incredible, it's only because it goes against all the conventional wisdom, but trust me, the conventional wisdom is wrong. I use the machine regularly and I can tell you it's without question one of the hardest and most effective workouts you can do. It allows you to burn off fat and build strength faster than anything else you can possibly do without leaving your house. You can find out more about the Xiser on my website, www.jonnybowden.com, under "four-minute exercise."

The fact that interval training is the most effective workout for fat loss shouldn't dissuade you from doing other things you enjoy, like hiking, tennis, Pilates, or running. And it certainly shouldn't dissuade you from lifting weights, which shapes your body, tones your muscles, and helps you burn more calories when you're at rest.

But for fat burning exercise, there's nothing that can compare to interval training. Make the switch now, and see what happens.

that exceeds your heart's capacity," he says. Sears believes that short bursts of high-intensity exercise create not just a reserve for your heart, but a hormonal environment conducive to fat loss.

If you still doubt this, ask yourself when you last saw a flabby sprinter. Flabby marathoner? Maybe. Sprinter? Never.

You can start PACE with an easy, ten-minute program. After warming up, spend one minute working hard enough to break a sweat and give your heart and lungs a challenge. Then slow down and let your heart rate recover for another minute. Repeat. Alternate one minute of exertion with one minute of recovery five times, for a total of 10 minutes. It's a great way to start interval training and really begin to lose the fat.

And your heart will thank you for it at the same time.

Yeast Infections

Prevent this Problem with This Combo Cure

THERE'S A FUNGUS AMONG US. And its name is Candida albicans. Also known as candida vaginitis, candidiasis, thrush, and "that-annoying-itch-that-is-making-me crazy," yeast infections are just not fun.

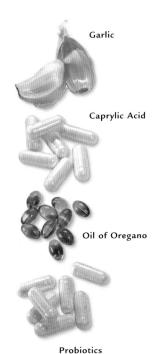

Garlic

Caprylic Acid

Oil of Oregano

Probiotics

They are an overgrowth of the Candida albicans bacteria and are one of the most common reasons women consult health-care professionals. But if you're thinking we're just talking "female problems," think again. A yeast infection may sound like girl talk, but the mischief done by Candida albicans goes way beyond that most obvious of syndromes. That mischief affects both men and women, and it's hardly limited to private parts. And it's serious.

A Gut Course in Ecology

Your gut, which is one of the most important and complex systems in the body and which Michael Gershon, M.D., aptly nicknamed "the second brain," is really akin to a complex ecological system. Think of it as a garden, populated by all sorts of beautiful flowers but plagued by annoying little weeds. If you keep those weeds in check, you've got a gorgeous garden. If you ignore them, they'll take over the garden, squeeze out the roots of the flowers, and leave you with something that looks like the lawn in Nightmare on Elm Street.

The flowers in that garden are analogous to the "good" bacteria in your gut. Collectively known as probiotics, these include such beneficial species as Bifidobacterium bifidum and Lactobacillus acidophilus. But that gut garden of yours also has its weeds—chief among them, Candida albicans. When the ecology gets out of balance, candida grows and multiplies like weeds (or rabbits). While a vaginal yeast infection is one common symptom of that, it's far from the only damage yeast can do. Yeast can actually travel throughout the body and become a systemic infection, producing symptoms both mental and physical. And candida, being a living organism, produces waste products that can be allergenic for some people. Simply put, an overgrowth of candida is not your friend.

So how does this imbalance happen in the first place? Let's start with candida's favorite food: sugar. Yeast thrives on sugar. Loves the stuff. Processed carbohydrates like breads and cereal are like "Miracle-Gro" for yeasty bugs.

Next, there are antibiotics, also known as candida's best friend. Why? Because, like a powerful weed killer that also kills your roses, antibiotics kill everything, making it even easier for candida to pop back up and overtake the farm. (Just like in your garden, it's easier for the weeds to come back than the roses.) Anyone on antibiotics for more than two weeks is at increased risk for an overgrowth of candida. Oral contraceptives, alcohol, caffeine, and immune suppressant medications (including corticosteroids) add to the problem. Put a high-sugar diet together with a course of antibiotics and you can pretty much guarantee you've got a serious candida problem.

It's a particularly insidious problem to have. Only in some cases are the symptoms localized and obvious—a vaginal yeast infection, for example, or a case of thrush, which is an overgrowth in the mouth. Most of the time the symptoms are general and somewhat ambiguous. You could experience anything from brain fog to fatigue to GI distress, rashes, hives, skin problems, or sinus infections—the connection to candida can be elusive. With such a wide range of diffuse symptoms, most people have no idea that they're infected with the little bugs. (One tip-off: Check under your toenails. If there's a fungus there, there's a good likelihood you've got yeast in your system.)

How Does Your Garden Grow?

What to do, what to do?

First thing is, you want to send some reinforcements for the good bacteria in your gut. Start with supplements of probiotics. These guys live in the small and large intestine and happily make vitamins for us, while keeping the overgrowth of the bad bugs in check. They boost the immune system and increase resistance to infection. Lactobacillus in particular is a species of friendly bacteria that is an integral part of normal vaginal flora; consider it a guard dog for candida overgrowth.

Probiotics offer a baker's dozen of health benefits. Remember that without a healthy, optimally functioning gut you can't properly absorb and utilize nutrients, so in a real sense a gut well tended to is the foundation of good health. Probiotics also have been shown to help prevent diarrhea and eczema, support the immune system, and reduce the frequency of the common cold.

Yogurt is the traditional source of beneficial bacteria; however, different brands of yogurt can vary greatly in their bacterial strain and potency. Look for something on the label that says "contains active cultures." Not "made from active cultures" because there may have been some living bacteria in the mix at one time, but heat and processing often kills them, so you want one that actually contains active cultures, not just one that had them long ago. (And by the way, the only thing "frozen yogurt" has in common with real yogurt that contains probiotics is that they're both white.) I'm also a big fan of kefir (fermented milk), goat's milk yogurt, and Greek-style yogurt. And I'm not a big fan of the no-fat kind, which contains more sugar than the regular varieties.

Probiotics are also available in supplement form, in both capsule and powder. They're alive, so refrigerate them for best results.

Starve the Critters: The Anti-Yeast Diet

If you want to get rid of yeast, you have to starve them. And that means not giving them their favorite food: sugar. Remember, yeast thrives in a sweet, carbo-loaded environment.

The best "anti-yeast" diets look like some version of the Atkins diet, at least for the first few weeks: no sugar, no processed carbs (grains, pastas, breads, and cereal products), no alcohol, vinegar, fruits, aged cheeses, peanuts, melons, and soy products, at least not in the beginning. Sorry to say, but beer is quite simply an infusion of yeast, so stay away. (Actually, except for the "no-fruit" rule, an anti-yeast diet is a pretty healthy way to eat. After you've gotten rid of them, you can always add back stuff, especially the fruit.) Here are some suggestions for your anti-yeast arsenal.

Coconut Oil. If you read my previous book, *The 150 Healthiest Foods on Earth*, you know I am an unabashed fan of coconut oil, one of nature's leading antifungal foods. It contains medium-chain fatty acids that help the body eliminate yeast. As a cooking oil, it is unmatched in its ability to tolerate a wide range of heat without burning or scorching. For those with systemic yeast overgrowth, ingesting 2 to 4 tablespoons of coconut oil daily is very beneficial.

Caprylic Acid. Caprylic acid is one of the fatty acids found in coconut oil and is also available as a separate supplement. Nutritionists and natural health practitioners have relied on it for years as a dependable yeast slayer. Its antifungal effect has been demonstrated in clinical trials. Though the exact

WORTH KNOWING

If you're mainly concerned with the more localized and specific form of a yeast problem, the common vaginal yeast infection, you can consider adding a douche to the natural prescription (above). Remember that the vaginal yeast infection is just one manifestation of candida, so it's a good idea not to skip the dietary and supplement recommendations. That said, a douche of one of the following may be a nice addition to the program. According to my associates, nutritionists Suzanne Copp, M.S., and Susan Mudd, M.S., C.N.S., these are all effective, so choose one that appeals to you and give it a try:

Boric acid: Studies show the effectiveness of boric acid as a douche is very high, especially in women with chronic resistant yeast infections. One study with 100 women showed a 98 percent success rate with this condition. Boric acid suppositories, containing 600 mg of boric acid, have been used successfully as a treatment for vaginal yeast infections. The suppositories were inserted vaginally twice a day for two weeks, then continued for an additional two weeks if necessary. Boric acid should never be swallowed.

Garlic: Insert a garlic clove into the vagina in the morning and an acidophilus capsule in the evening for three to seven days.

Combo douche: Prepare a retention douche (in which the preparation of substances stays in the vagina and is not flushed out) with equal parts bentonite clay, pau d'arco tea, yogurt, tea tree oil, and goldenseal, and douche two times a day for seven to ten days.

Tea tree oil: Soak a tampon with diluted tea tree oil and keep it in the vagina overnight.

mechanism of its action against yeast isn't completely understood, we think it penetrates and destabilizes the yeast cell walls. Caprylic acid is absorbed very rapidly, so capsules should be enteric coated or timed release for best results

Garlic. Known as Russian penicillin, garlic is considered nature's premier antibiotic and antifungal, which makes it a perfect adversary for candida. It's like a stealth smart-bomb—it's effective against bad bacteria and yeast but leaves the body's normal, friendly bugs unharmed. Several studies demonstrate the power of garlic to combat candida, with some showing garlic to be more powerful than nystatin, gentian violet, and other standard antifungal agents.

Oil of Oregano. Oil of oregano has been used for years in the treatment of candida, and studies have demonstrated the effectiveness of oils in the destruction of candida. In fact, oil of oregano is such a powerful antimicrobial that it prompted one physician, Cass Ingram, D.O., to write a book on it, aptly titled *The Cure Is in the Cupboard*. Wild oregano as well as extracts of olive leaf are recognized for their potent antifungal, antibacterial, antiviral, and antiparasitic properties. Oregano can be made into a tea by steeping 1 to 2 teaspoons of the dried herb in hot water for ten minutes. You can drink the tea three times a day. You can also take both oil of oregano and olive oil extract as supplements. Note: If you're pregnant, don't use oil of oregano, as it may induce miscarriage.

Natural Prescription for Yeast Infections

Probiotics: 10 to 30 billion bacteria, in capsule or powder form. Take with food.

Diet: Eliminate sugar, alcohol, bread, moldy foods like cheeses, melons, and pistachios.

Caprylic acid: 500 to 2,000 mg, three times a day, with meals.

Oil of oregano: 250 to 500 mg, three times a day. Or drink oregano tea three times a day.

Garlic: 600 to 900 mg per day, in divided doses

FOR ADDED EFFECTIVENESS:

Boric acid suppositories: Insert into vagina. Never drink boric acid.

ALSO RECOMMENDED:

Pau d'arco tea: Steep for five minutes and drink three times a day. A natural antifungal agent.

Note: All the dosages above are daily and in pill or capsule form unless otherwise noted.

ACKNOWLEDGMENTS

Writing a book like this requires many things, but chief among them is an amazing Rolodex (okay, make that a Palm Pilot). I've got one of the best. Even though I don't always make use of every name that's in it for every book I write, the fact that these folks are there and available to me, and that I know they will—and have, and do—give generously of their time and their information, makes it much easier to proceed with a project like this. So for all of those who contributed your time and energy so willingly and graciously, I thank you enormously.

Stephen Sinatra, M.D., read and critiqued the "Awesome Foursome" chapter on heart disease. Mark Houston, M.D., M.S., gave me his always invaluable input on the hypertension section. Acupuncturist Cindy Lawrence, LAc, was essential for the section on acupuncture and fertility, ditto Matthew Mannino, D.O., for the section on chiropractic and back pain. Kathryn Shafer, Ph.D., helped enormously with the section on image therapy for asthma, as did Bill Flocco with the section on PMS and reflexology, and Harry Preuss, M.D. with the section on weight loss supplements. Bert Berkson, M.D., Ph.D., gave generously of his time and was essential to the section on hepatitis C. Joe Brasco, M.D. ("GI Joe") was as always a rich source of information on everything to do with gastrointestinal illness. Robbie Dunton, M.D., was kind enough to proofread the EMDR chapter, and Joan Mathews-Larson, Ph.D. could not have been more gracious in offering her input for the section on addiction. Others who contributed their time, valuable info, and input include Daniel Amen, M.D., Hyla Cass, M.D., Shari Lieberman, Ph.D., Parris Kidd, Ph.D., Andrew Rubman, N.D., Robert Portman, Ph.D., and Al Sears, M.D.

And for all my "rolodex regulars" who I didn't call on this time, I still appreciate you for being there in case I needed you: Jacob Teitelbaum, M.D., Timothy Birdsall, N.D., David Ludwig, M.D., Ph.D., Evelyn Tribole, M.S., R.D., Regina

Wilshire, N.D., David Leonardi, M.D., C. Leigh Broadhurst, Ph.D., Dharma Singh Khalsa, M.D., Jeffrey Bland, Ph.D., Alan Gaby, M.D., Elson Haas, M.D., Ann Louise Gittleman, Ph.D., Barry Sears, Ph.D., Fred Pescatore, M.D., Colette Heimowitz, M.S., Oz Garcia, John Abramson, M.D., Robert Crayhon, M.S., Sonja Petterson, N.D., Charles Poliquin, Richard Firshein, D.O., J. J. Virgin, Ph.D., Linda Lizotte, R.D., David Brady, N.D., Esther Blum, R.D., Liz Neporent, M.S., C.S.C.S., Michael Eades, M.D., Mary Dan Eades, M.D., Cathy Wong, N.D., Karl Knopf, Ph.D., Kilmer McCully, M.D., Ron Rosdale, M.D., Robert Roundtree, M.D., Walter Willett, M.D., Ph.D., Mehmet Oz, M.D., and Christiane Northrup, M.D. And don't think you'll get away without a call next time.

I'd also like to thank and acknowledge the most comprehensive and thorough database on natural medicine in the world, The Natural Standard, whose staff generously allowed me access to their subscription-only website, www.natural-standard.com. Their assistance was invaluable and was greatly appreciated, and I recommend them highly. And each year, Tod Cooperman, M.D., is kind enough to give me free access to www.consumerlab.com, for which I am grateful as well.

But wait, there's more!

I've said it before and I'll say it again—I have the best literary agent in the world. Coleen O'Shea nurtures, protects, fertilizes, and germinates ideas and projects and then goes out and makes them happen. And takes my calls at all hours of the night. She's an endless source of support. I'm lucky to have her.

My editor, Cara Connors, did the best thing in the world an editor can do for a writer: She "got" me. And she edited in the smartest way possible for an editor who has to deal with a writer (like me) who doesn't like being edited—selectively and judiciously and intelligently, making every change count and winning my respect and admiration in the process. Great job.

My publishers, Will Kiester and Ken Fund, who believe in the Jonny Bowden brand, and the amazing editors, designers, and copyeditors at Fair Winds Press—especially John Gettings, Tiffany Hill, and Dutton and Sherman Design, and Megan Cooney who make each of my books look so gorgeous I almost can't believe it.

My Web designer, Christopher Loch, who designed my website, made it beautiful, and best of all, has made it possible for me not to ever have to learn anything about html. You can contact him at www.whatismysecret.com, but don't even think about trying to steal him away from me.

The many teachers who continue to inspire me on a daily basis—Jack Canfield, Mark Victor Hanson, Les Brown, Armand Moran, and especially to my good friends, Alex Mandossian and T. Harv Eker.

To Werner Erhard, who started me on a path that changed my life and continues to influence me—almost forty years later—to this day. Wherever you are, I love you.

My editors at my "day jobs" who keep me up to my neck in interesting and challenging projects when I'm not writing books—especially Nicole Wise and Sarah Hiner at Boardroom, Colette Heimowitz at Atkins Nutritionals, Kalia Donner at Remedy, Lyle Hurd at Total Health, Adam Campbell and Jeff O'Connell at Men's Health, and Tanya Mancini and the gang at America Online. All the folks at Greenstone media—especially Heather Cohen—deserve a special smile. Mo Gaffney, Shana Wride, and Sally Jesse Raphael always make my radio appearances a pleasure.

My publicists, Mary Aarons at Fair Winds Press, and Melissa McNeese and Leslie McClure, for doing such a great job of getting me out there.

Hollywood stars have their stylists, their hair people, and their makeup artists to make them look as good as they do when they walk down the red carpet. I, on the other hand, have "The Sues."

Suzanne Copp and Susan Mudd are two of the smartest and most dedicated nutritionists I know, and I could not have written this book—at least and have it finished in less than a decade—without their tireless support.

Suzanne Copp, M.S., is a clinical nutritionist who has maintained a private practice in Connecticut that focuses on health conditions such as weight loss, women's issues, hypoglycemia, diabetes, gastrointestinal ailments, and eating disorders. A former adjunct professor in the nutrition department at the prestigious University of Bridgeport, she now works as a consultant for Crayhon Research focusing on writing and editorial projects.

Susan Mudd, M.S., C.N.S., is a clinical nutritionist practicing in Gaithersburg, Maryland. She maintains a busy client practice, is a sought-after speaker and consultant and writes a monthly column called "Edible Insights." She is also a licensed provider of "Shapedown," a program focused on child and adolescent obesity counseling. I am eternally grateful for their enormous contributions to this project.

My writing style would not be what it is without the input of an eclectic group of writers, some of whom have delighted me since I was old enough to read (Harold Pinter, Tennessee Williams) others of whom I discovered later but whose work has shaped mine as surely as if I had sat at their feet in an imaginary classroom. One in particular stands out in this eclectic group, William Goldman. I would not be the writer I am today if William Goldman hadn't enriched my life with his every written word. He's simply not capable of writing anything bad. Thanks are also due to the late Ed McBain (Evan Hunter). And to the best science writer in America, Robert Sapolsky, whose writing serves as a model for anyone wanting to educate and entertain at the same time. No one alive does it better.

My love and gratitude goes out to my family—Jeffrey Bowden, Nancy Fiedler, Pace Bowden, and Cadence Bowden for, well, being my family. Which can't always be easy, hard as that is to believe. And as always, to the people and animals I love who make my life wonderful: Susan Wood and Christopher Duncan, my partner-in-crime Jackie (Sky London) Balough, my brother Peter Breger, my sisters Randy Graff and Lauree Dash, Kimberly Wright the Sushi Goddess, my lifelong friend Jeanette Lee Bessinger, Scott Ellis, Ron Ellison, Dr. Richard Lewis, Gina Lombardi and Kevin Sizemore, Anita Waxman, Diane Lederman, Oz Garcia (when I can find him), Billy Stritch, Liz Neporent, Zack Kleinmann, Marlon Reveche, Oliver Becaud, Jennifer Schneider, and Leslie.

And to Howard, Robin, Gary, Fred, and Artie for continuing to make me smile every single morning since 1995.

And to Woodstock and Emily the Second for whom I am grateful on a daily basis.

And of course, to Anja, my muse, the love of my life … in all ways and for always.

ABOUT THE AUTHOR

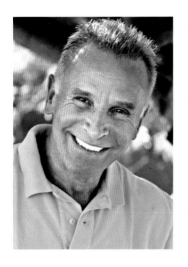

Jonny Bowden, Ph.D., C.N.S., a board-certified nutritionist, is a nationally known expert on nutrition, weight loss, and health. A former member of the editorial advisory board of *Men's Health* magazine and a health columnist for America Online, he's also written or contributed to articles for dozens of national publications (print and online) including the *New York Times*, *Wall Street Journal*, *Forbes*, *Time*, *Oxygen*, *Marie Claire*, *W*, *Remedy*, *Diabetes Focus*, *Cosmopolitan*, *Family Circle*, *Self*, *Fitness*, *Prevention*, and *Shape*. He is the author of the award-winning *Living Low Carb: Controlled Carbohydrate Eating for Long-Term Weight Loss*, *The Most Effective Ways to Live Longer*, *The 150 Most Effective Ways to Boost Your Energy*, and his acclaimed signature bestseller, *The 150 Healthiest Foods on Earth*. A popular, dynamic, and much sought-after speaker, he's appeared on CNN, Fox News, MSNBC, ABC, NBC, and CBS, and speaks frequently around the country. He lives in Southern California.

INDEX

borage oil, 108
boric acid, 241, 243
Bortz, Walter, 15
boswellia, 182
BPH. *See* benign prostatic hyperplasia (BPH)
brain
    exercise and, 44
    mental exercise and, 41, 44
    nutrients for better functioning of, 27–40
    nutrition, 27
    protecting your, 24–25
    size, 26
    stress and, 42–43, 193
Brasco, Joe, 11, 179–180
Bratman, Steven, 30, 37, 89
Bray, George, 69–70
breathing exercises, 43
Brown, Richard P., 191
Bryan, Nathan, 162–163
BSP, 62, 63
butterbur, 199, 204, 205, 206
B vitamins, 35–36, 54. *See also specific vitamins*

C
cabbage juice, 229
caffeine, 131
calcium, 156, 222–223
calcium oxalate, 187–188
Candida albicans, 73, 236–243
caprylic acid, 240, 242, 243
carbohydrates, acne and, 19–20
cardiovascular disease, 116–125
carnitine, 28, 29, 117–121, 125
cataracts, 198
catecholamines, 124
Cathcart, Robert, 139
Celebrex, 58, 59, 113
celery, 158
chamomile, 108
charcoal, 73, 75
chasteberry, 224, 225
cherries, 113–114
childhood asthma, 128
Chinese herbs, 186
chlorophyll, 73, 74, 137
chocolate, 131, 201
cholesterol, 124

chondroitin, 57–60, 63
Chopra, Deepak, 109
chromium, 94–96, 100, 213, 214
cinnamon, 100, 101–102
coconut oil, 137–138, 179, 240
coenzyme Q10, 31, 116–121, 125, 155, 199, 203, 205
cognitive decline, 24, 27, 36–40, 44–45
colds, 164–166
cold sores, 143–147
combo douche, 241
congestive heart failure, 116–117, 118
contact dermatitis, 102
Cordina, Loren, 18–19
coriander, 74
COX-2 inhibitors, 58, 113–114
Craig, Gary, 109, 110–111
cravings, 80–83
C-reactive protein, 123
Crohn's disease, 176–182
cruciferous vegetables, 150
cumin, 74
cysteine, 198

D
dairy, 50, 106, 179–180
dandelion root, 140, 141
DASH diet, 153–158
deglycyrrhizinated licorice (DGL), 229
delta-6-desaturase, 106–107
dementia, 25–26, 29, 35–38, 44
depression, 52, 83–92
detoxification, 73, 137
DHA (docosahexaenoic acid), 40
DHT (dihydrotestosterone), 22–23, 77
diabetes, 92–102
diabetic retinopathy, 194
diet
    acne and, 16–21
    aging and, 31
    anti-yeast, 73, 240, 242
    bad breath and, 73–74
    brain and, 27
    cognitive decline and, 39–40
    DASH, 153–158
    eczema and, 104–106
    elimination, 48–50, 52, 105–106

magnesium, 125
    for aging complications, 31, 43
    for anxiety, 55
    for asthma, 69, 71
    for diabetes, 96–97, 100
    for heart disease, 120–121, 124
    for hypertension, 156, 158
    for kidney stones, 188–189
    for migraines, 199, 203, 204, 205
    for PMS, 221
mast cells, 67
Mathews-Larson, Joan, 82
McCleary, Larry, 25
McDougall, John, 16
meat, 20, 21
meditation, 43
melatonin, 85, 183
membranes, 29–30
memory loss, 24, 38
menopause, 148–151
menstrual irregularities, 209
mental exercise, 41, 44
metabolic arthritis, 112–115
metabolic syndrome, 92–102, 208
metaformin, 212, 213
methyl sulfonylmethane (MSM), 61, 63
migraines, 52, 199–206
mild cognitive impairment (MCI), 25–26
milk, 20, 131–132
milk thistle, 138–139, 141
mint, 74
mitochondria, 27–28, 34, 117
mitochondrial dysfunction, 27–28
multiple sclerosis, 38
multiple vitamin, 31
multivitamin, 197, 198
Murray, Michael, 21, 181
myelin sheath, 35

N

N-acetyl-cysteine (NAC), 139, 141
nasal decongestants, 46
natural cures
    effectiveness of, 11–12
    research on, 13–14
neominophagen, 140
nettles, 78, 79

neurochemicals, 112
neurons, 26, 39–40
neurotransmitters, 38
niacin, 40
Nieman, David, 66–67
nitric oxide (NO), 161, 162–163
nonsteroidal anti-inflammatory drugs (NSAIDs), 228–230
norepinephrine, 85
Northrup, Christiane, 149
nutrition, 27. See also diet
nutritional medicine, 9–10

O

obsessive-compulsive disorder (OCD), 55, 184–185
oil of oregano, 73, 75, 242, 243
olive leaf complex, 168–170
omega-3 fatty acids
    for aging complications, 31, 40
    anti-inflammatory properties of, 123
    for arthritis, 59, 61–63
    for depression, 90
    for diabetes, 100, 101
    heart disease and, 121–123
    hypertension and, 156
    macular degeneration and, 197–198
omega-6 fatty acids, 107
osteoarthritis, 56–63
ovarian cysts, 209–210
oxalate, 187–188
oxidative stress, 70, 98
oxytocin, 43

P

PACE program, 234, 236
Packer, Lester, 138
paleo diet, 12, 19, 21, 22
panic disorders, 55
Parkinson's disease, 38
parsley, 74
pau d'arco tea, 243
peelu, 74
pepsin, 227
peripheral artery disease, 118
peripheral neuropathy, 98
Perlmutter, David, 28, 29, 34
Pert, Candace, 109

Peruvian ginseng, 160–161
Petterson, Sonja, 10
phosphatidylcholine, 141–142
phosphatidylserine (PS), 29–30, 31
phospholipids, 29, 32
plant sterols, 147
pollen, 46
polycystic ovary syndrome (PCOS), 207–214
polyphenols, 40, 66, 168–169
pomegranate juice, 124–125
post-traumatic stress disorder (PTSD), 215–220
potassium, 156, 158
pregnancy, 87
premenstrual syndrome (PMS), 220–225
Preuss, Harry, 94
probiotics, 72, 75, 103, 107–108, 132–134, 181,
    182, 229, 239, 240, 243
processed foods, 21
progesterone, 148
prolactin, 87
prostaglandins, 106
prostate, 76–79
PSA (prostate-specific antigen), 77
pumpkin seeds, 78, 189
pygeum, 78, 79

Q
qi, 172–173
quercetin, 47, 51, 66–67, 69

R
Reishi mushrooms, 140–141
Remifemin, 149
research, on natural cures, 13–14
Reston, James, 171
resveratrol, 158
rhodiola rosea, 190–193
riboflavin, 199, 203, 204, 205
ribose, 119–120, 122, 125
Ritchason, Jack, 170
Roberts, James, 119
Robins, Eric, 111, 112
rotation diet, 48–50, 52
Rubman, Andrew, 227
rule of thirds, 11–12, 180

S
Sahelian, Ray, 54
SAMe, 89–92, 140
saw palmetto, 21–23, 77, 79
Schaeffer, O., 18
schizophrenia, 38
scopolamine amnesia, 32–33
Sears, Al, 234, 236
Sears, Barry, 93
seasonal allergies, 45–48, 51
sebum, 17, 21–22
Seddon, Johanna, 198
selenium, 69, 70, 108, 136, 138, 141
self-healing, 10–11
senior moments, 24
serotonin, 43, 54, 84–86, 184–185
serotonin selective reuptake inhibitors (SSRIs),
    84–85
Shapiro, Francine, 215–217
Shapiro, William, 177
shea nut oil, 58, 62, 63
shiitake mushrooms, 140–141
side effects, 12
signaling, 40
silymarin, 141
Sinatra, Stephen, 117, 119–120
Sit and Be Fit program, 62
sleep disorders, 183–186
smoking, 134, 158
sodium, 153–154, 155
soft drinks, 115, 188
soy, 150, 151
Specific Carbohydrate Diet (SCD), 178–179
spinach, 40
standard American diet (SAD), 153
Starbuck, Jaimison, 47–48
stinging nettles, 51, 78, 79
St. John's wort, 86–90, 148
Stoll, Andrew, 123
stomach acid, 69–70, 72, 127–131, 134, 227
strawberries, 40
stress
    allergies and, 68
    asthma and, 68
    brain and, 42–43, 193
    cardiovascular health and, 124

herpes and, 145
infertility and, 174
magnesium and, 121, 124
PCOS and, 212
weight gain and, 42
stress fatigue, 190–193
sugar, 50, 73, 106, 202, 208, 214, 238
sugar cravings, 80–83
sulfur, 61
sylmarin, 136

T

tai chi, 62
Talanian, Jason, 232–234
taurine, 125, 224
tea tree oil, 147, 241
Teitelbaum, Jacob, 54, 122
testosterone, 19, 21–22, 77
theanine, 53–55
theobromine, 131
traditional Chinese medicine (TCM), 171–172
trauma, 215–220
triglycerides, 121–122
trimethylglycine (TMG), 133
tryptophan, 85
turmeric, 137
type 1 diabetes, 95
type 2 diabetes, 92–102
tyrmaines, 201

U

ulcerative colitis, 176–182
ulcers, 226–230
uric acid, 112–113, 187
urination, frequent, 76

V

vaginal yeast infection, 241. *See also* yeast infections
vegetable juice, 73–74, 138
vinpocentine, 31, 34–35
Vioxx, 58
vision issues, 194–198
vitamin B2, 203, 204, 205
vitamin B6, 36, 54, 69, 71, 85, 188–189, 221
vitamin B12, 35–36, 54, 129
vitamin C, 31, 51, 69, 70, 100, 139, 147, 156, 195

vitamin D, 181, 182, 222–223
vitamin E, 31, 125, 140, 147, 150, 195
vitex, 224, 225

W

water, 132
water aerobics, 62
weight gain, 42, 208, 209
weight loss, 213–214, 231–236
wheat, 50, 106
wheatgrass juice, 137
whey protein powder, 139, 141, 156
white willow bark, 205
whole foods, 73
Williams, Roger, 80–81
witch hazel, 108
Wright, Jonathan, 64, 127–128, 130

X

Xiser, 235

Y

yeast, 73
yeast infections, 236–243
yin and yang, 172
yogurt, 239

Z

zeaxanthin, 196–197
ZEN supplement, 54
zinc, 78–79, 100, 108, 163–168, 195, 198
zinc carnosine, 226–230